How To Do A Color Analysis

10 Steps to Completing the Perfect Color Analysis

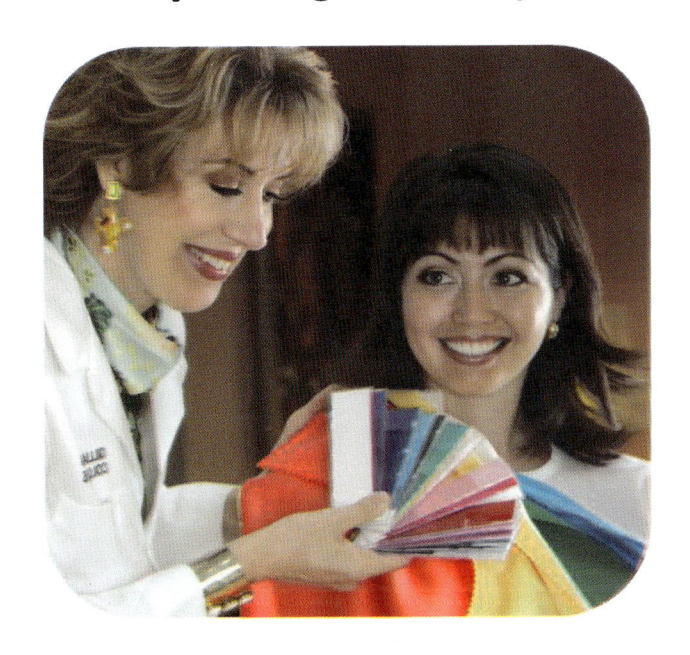

By Gillian Armour, AICI CIP

First Printing, April 2011

10 9 8 7 6 5 4 3 2 1

Copyright ©2011 GILLIAN ARMOUR DESIGN LLC
All rights reserved.

ISBN-13: 978-1461028116

ISBN-10: 1461028116

Printed in the United States of America.
Set in Calibri.

All Images ©Gillian Armour
Wikipedia Public Domain Images as Indicated

Without limiting the rights under copyright reserved above, no part of this publication may be reproduced, stored in or introduced into a retrieval system, or transmitted, in any form, or by any means (electronic, mechanical, photocopying, recording or otherwise), without the prior written permission of both the copyright owner and the publisher of this book.

Note:
The scanning, uploading, and distribution of this book via the Internet or via any other means without the permission of the publisher is illegal and punishable by law. Please purchase only authorized electronic editions, and do not participate in or encourage electronic piracy of copyrighted materials. Your support of the author's rights is appreciated.

Introduction		p 5
Chapter 1	What is Color?	p 11
Chapter 2	History of Color Analysis	p 23
Chapter 3	Ten Steps to a Perfect Color Analysis	p 31
	Step One - Prepare	p 37
	Step Two - Client Interview	p 41
	Step Three - Painting Skin Tone	p 47
	Step Four - Draping	p 49
	Step Five - Testing Hair Color	p 53
	Step Six - Analyze Color Temperature	p 55
	Step Seven - Color, Print, Texture Tests	p 59
	Step Eight - Creating Color Fans	p 69
	Step Nine - Makeup	p 71
	Step Ten - Optional Services	p 73
Chapter 4	Marketing Your Business	p 75
	Setting Your Fees	p 81
Chapter 5	Articles and Forms for Clients	p 83
TRAINING AND CERTIFICATION		p 97
ABOUT		p 105

Introduction

"Music is equipped with a system by which it defines each sound in terms of its pitch, intensify, and duration, without dragging in loose allusions to the endlessly varying sounds of nature. So should color be supplied with an appropriate system, based on the hue, value, and chroma of our sensations, and not attempting to describe them by the indefinite and varying colors of natural objects." *Albert Munsell (1858-1915)*

As a successful color analyst, I've had the great pleasure of introducing hundreds of clients to the joys of color. Clients discovering their best colors undergo irreversible transformations. They go from dressing "yeow" to dressing "wow." I get such joy watching this transformation happen and you will too.

I have earned several color analysis certifications in specializations ranging from ethnic skin tone to eight season color analysis. I have practiced color analysis for years and successfully analyzed hundreds of clients. The systems I used in the past were based on the 4, 8 or 12 seasonal color analysis methods (Spring Summer, Autumn, Winter/ low-contrast, high-contrast/ deep, light, bright, clear etc. and etc.). These seasonal systems were quite often confusing for my clients and students - and so one day I asked myself "Why are seasonal terms used to identify a person's coloring when in nature there are only **TWO** underlying degrees of temperature (warm and cool)?" I wondered what it would be like to have a simple way to analyze clients, one that would give them a broad range of color options to wear.

And, because I wanted a system that was easy to teach and effective to implement, I simplified my color analysis method into a system I call **2D/3D=EZ**© (two degrees of color in three dimensional views equals easy!) in the hope that students can readily understand how color is analyzed and can better communicate that with their clients. My system simplifies color analysis into degrees of temperature: **WARM** and **COOL**. After all, there are only two color degrees in nature and in the world of color. A client is either warm or cool based in her skin tone. Simple. Or is it?

Can You Tell?

Look at the photos on the left side of this page. Can you tell if the person is a cool skin tone? Now look at the same person pictured in the right column. Do you still think they are a cool skin tone or a warm skin tone?

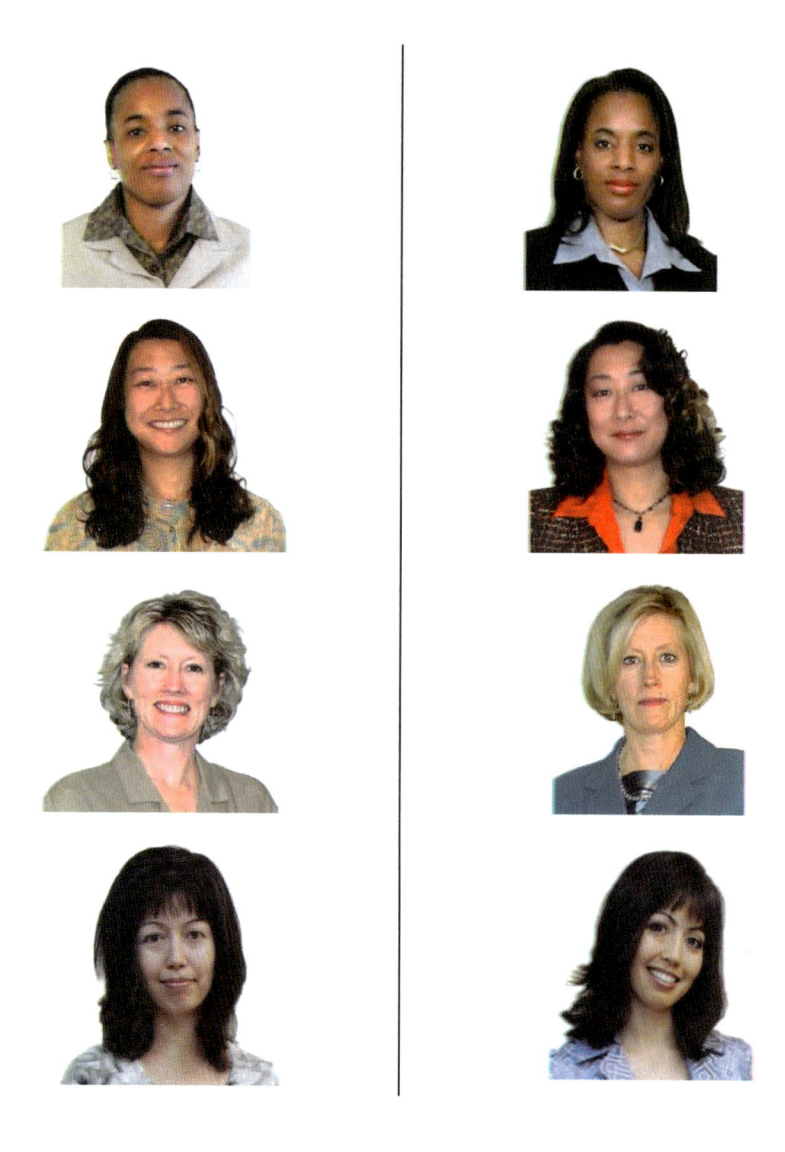

Are you uncertain? Confused? Unsure? Even bewildered? My guess is you are and, as you know, your clients will be just as confused when they come to you for help. (*see next page for answers*)

In this book I will distill into ten simple steps a method of color analyzing that is proven successful AND easy for you, as the consultant, to follow.

By reading this book and learning these ten steps you will learn:

- How to precisely define a clients underlying skin coloring.
- To successfully determine cool or warm dimensions in skin coloration.
- Accurately analyze low, medium or high degree (contrast) in skin color.
- How to conduct an initial color consultation with new clients.
- Business basics such as marketing, targeting clients and developing strategic alliances.

There are many color analysis professionals who have developed their own successful system of color analysis and stay true to their own methodology and theory; so as not to confuse I purposely do NOT refer much to other color analysis creators and their systems in this book other than in the section on the history of color analysis.

However, if you are reading this and seeking a color analysis, be sure to choose certified and experienced color analysts only. I say this because I get a lot of feedback from frustrated clients who have been incorrectly analyzed by so called "professional color analysts" who are neither certified nor experienced.

Before detailing the ten steps of a color analysis, I would like to stress that this book is a basic guideline for consultants wishing to add this service to their menu of image consulting offerings. These steps are tried and true but they are not a substitute for hands-on, in-person training. I highly recommend that this book be a starting point for you in your process toward becoming a certified color analyst. It has been my experience that the nuances of color and the appropriate ones for clients are best discovered with practice and a good teacher. At the back of this book you will find information detailing the training programs available to you here at Fashion Image Institute.

Answers to page 6 **Cool or Warm?**: 1)cool 2) warm 3) cool 4) cool

Understanding the Power of Color

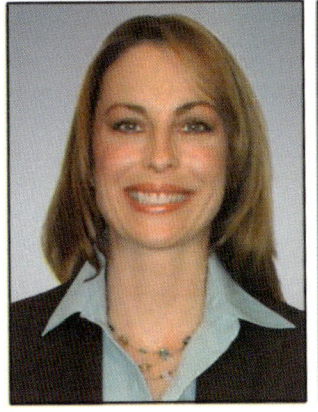

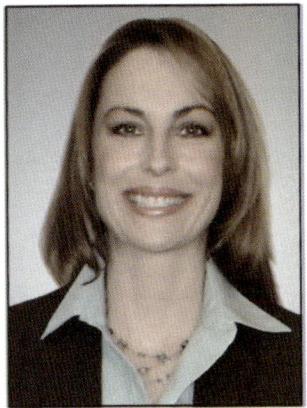

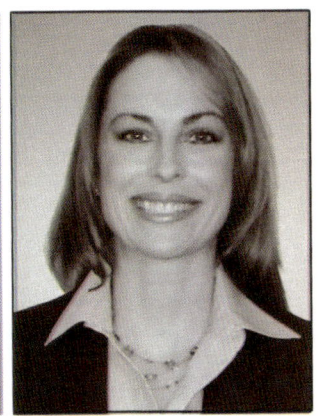

Color is one of the most effective ways to say to the world, "Hey, look at me." While it would be gauche indeed to walk into a room and command attention in such an obvious way, you can accomplish the same results more subtlety when you wear colors that reflect your personal coloring. Just as great artists have a favored palette of colors they work with repeatedly, each person has a unique combination of skin, hair, and eye colors that make up their personal color palette. Building your wardrobe around these colors will literally **make you more visible**.

Color has been described as a tool of attraction. The following exercise will help illustrate this point. Relax for a moment and imagine you are driving along a country road. As you are driving along the road you meet a shiny red sports car. Notice your response when you see the car. Next, imagine that a little further on you round a corner and see before you a field of blue lupine in full bloom. What is your response to the field of lupine? Even if you haven't been dreaming about buying a red sports car and even if lupine isn't your favorite flower, your attention would surely have been captured by the unexpected encounter with these vivid colors. Both of these examples illustrate how bold, vivid, or unexpected color attracts our attention.

Color also attracts our attention through repetition. In the same way that repeating a thought or phrase adds rhetorical emphasis, repeating colors from your personal palette in the clothing you wear, adds visual emphasis. It is the easy, effective, and most powerful way to literally make yourself more visible.

Once color has gotten our attention it continues to influence our perceptions. Color can actually help sharpen the focus of our attention. In much the same way adjusting the lens of a camera brings a photograph into focus, adjusting the colors you wear can bring your image into clearer focus. When you wear colors that are in harmony with your personal palette you become more memorable. People have an easier time seeing you and an easier time hearing what you have to say. Your ability to bring your gifts and talents into the world is heightened.

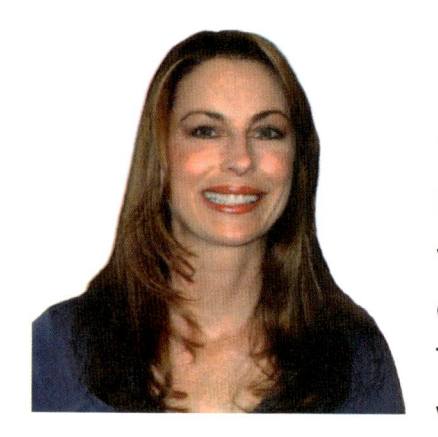

Ideally, we recommend that anyone who wants to polish their image work one-on-one with a certified image consultant. Such consultants are experts at helping you discover the color palette that reflects your personal coloring. When you work with an image consultant they can quickly identify your best colors. This is the surest, easiest way to heighten your visibility. But if that's not a practical solution for you, here are some guidelines you can follow that will help ensure you are making good choices on your own.

CH 1 What is Color?

"The system now to be considered portrays the three dimensions of color, and measures each by an appropriate scale. It does not rest upon the whim of an individual, but upon physical measurements made possible by special color apparatus. The results may be tested by anyone who comes to the problem with "a clear mind, a good eye, and a fair supply of patience."
Albert Munsell

Before you get good at color consulting you need to learn the foundational principles of color. In this chapter I touch on these principles so you have an understanding of what lies behind the advice you give your clients.

My explanations of color theory, color psychology, color properties and abilities are abbreviated in this book. I recommend you study further from the many color reference books available to you. You can contact me directly for my recommendations.

Simply put - color is the range, spectrum of tones and shades we see all around us. Wikipedia defines it as "the visual perceptual property corresponding in humans to the categories called *red*, *green*, *blue* and others. Color derives from the spectrum of light (distribution of light energy versus wavelength) interacting in the eye." The online dictionary also states that "the ability of the human eye to distinguish colors is based upon the varying sensitivity of different cells in the retina to the light of different wavelengths. The retina contains three types of color receptor cells, or cones."

Color has other definitions depending on physics, perception and association and as a category of study it is a rich field indeed. Many scientists have devoted their lives to the study of color; researching its wavelengths and spectrums. Philosophers and inventors from Aristotle to Sir Isaac Newton have mined its properties and identified aspects of color humans knew nothing about. Newton, in 1675, invented the color wheel and was the first in a long line of color analysts to identify how light created color.

Scientists have also discovered that our perception of color begins when a color enters the brain through the cones in the retina of the eye where they are then registered as brainwaves. From there different levels of color processing take place within the brain and colors are registered as distinct from each other.

"A dominant theory of color vision proposes that color information is transmitted out of the eye by three opponent channels, each constructed from the raw output of the cones: a red-green channel, a blue-yellow channel and a black-white channel. This theory has been supported by neurobiology, and accounts for the structure of our subjective color experience. Specifically, it explains why we cannot perceive a "reddish green" or "yellowish blue," and it predicts the color wheel: it is the collection of colors for which at least one of the two color channels measures a value at one of its extremes." Wikipedia Online Dictionary

Hue, Value And Chroma

"It may sound strange to say that color has three dimensions, but it is easily proved by the fact that each of them can be measured. Thus in the case of the boy's faded cap its redness or HUE is determined by one instrument; the amount of light in the red, which is its VALUE, and is found by another instrument; while still a third instrument determines the purity or CHROMA of the red." Albert Munsell

HUE = IS THE NAME OF A COLOR

A color's undertone - cool (blue based) or warm (yellow based). In painting and art color hue refers to a color's purity and is not diluted with white or black. It is the color in its original form - red, blue, yellow etc. Hue can also be defined as how we describe a dimension of a color - pinkish red, bluish purple etc.

VALUE = IS THE LIGHT OF THE COLOR

The depth of a color is usually described as "dark", "light" or "true." Value describes how light, bright, dark or deep a color is. For example, there are many shades of red but their value can be light red, bright red, deep red or dark red.

CHROMA = IS THE STRENGTH OF THE COLOR

The clarity of a color; pure, true, bright, vibrant, muted, dusty etc. The terms chromatic and monochromatic are also used to describe a color that contains a pure color (chromatic) or is dulled with another color (black or white) to appear washed out or muted (mono-chromatic). Adding black will mute the chroma of a color, adding white will brighten the chroma of a color.

It is true that in some color analysis systems skin-tones are defined by chroma (i.e.: vibrant spring, clear winter etc.) but it is not necessary to make a descriptive distinction when diagnosing cool or warm temperature.

Color Psychology

Color psychology, an extension of color analysis, is a valuable tool that is used in conjunction with the analysis of colors. In reality, the psychological connotation of a color has nothing to do with its effect upon the color of one's face or the results in the mirror. It is necessary to consider both the physical impact color has upon your appearance, and the impact a color has upon the unique persona that one projects to the world.

It is important to understand the psychological impact of the different colors in the color family so your client can use them to maximum effectiveness for any given occasion or purpose. As you will learn, certain color groups are more effective in certain situations. Here are a few examples:

The Best Colors to Wear for Business Meetings or Lunches (with colleagues or clients)
Black = power, strength, charisma.
Navy Blue = trustworthiness.
Royal Blue = sends out signals of goodwill.
Deep Gray = projects success and strength.
Camel or shades of Brown = appears non-threatening, stable, supportive and reliable.
Terra-cotta or brick = projects warmth and sensuality.
Blue Reds = indicate warmth, vitality.

Colors to Wear When Promoting or Selling a Product
True Blue or lighter shades of blue inspire trust.
Orange is friendly and appeals to all.
Yellow is cheerful and stimulating.
Blue based pinks calm and inspire others.

Colors of the Fashion Conscious
Lipstick Red = implies strength and authority.
Fuchsia = vivaciousness and dynamism.
Deep Purple = indicates creativity and artistic power.
Lilac = spiritual.
Muted and clear orange = warmth and earthiness.
Raspberry = to appear friendly and intelligent.
Celadon = calming and elegant.

Training Your Eye

We start to form color associations at a very young age. Sociologists have found that babies as young as 3 months old respond to colors. They can recognize primary colors of yellow, red and blue. It's not surprising that toys are manufactured in primary colors to stimulate young eyes and minds. M.H. Bornstein's 1976 study, *('The Categories of Hue In Infancy', M.H. Bornstein, W. Kessen and S. Weiskopf)*, found that infants can respond and recognize colors and hues of all types; preferring blues and purples over reds and yellows.

Artists can easily identify color and its many hues because they have been trained to do so. They have developed a critical eye - a way of seeing that takes practice and can be developed in any one of us. This book is obviously not designed to train an artist, BUT we do want you to learn how to develop your eye so you can give an accurate color analysis to your clients.

Take a look at the color wheel examples on the next page. Studying a color wheel will improve your eye toward identifying colors and their underlying temperatures of cool or warm.

A good rule of thumb to remember is that COOL colors have blue as their base and WARM colors have yellow. If you divide a color wheel in half you will notice that all the COOL colors are on one side and all the WARM on the other.

Now, take a closer look. Can you see that all the COOL colors have a slight blue tinge to them and the WARM a slight yellow tinge? That tinge is the undertone. Similar to what you will see in your clients eyes, hair and skin when you are doing an analysis.

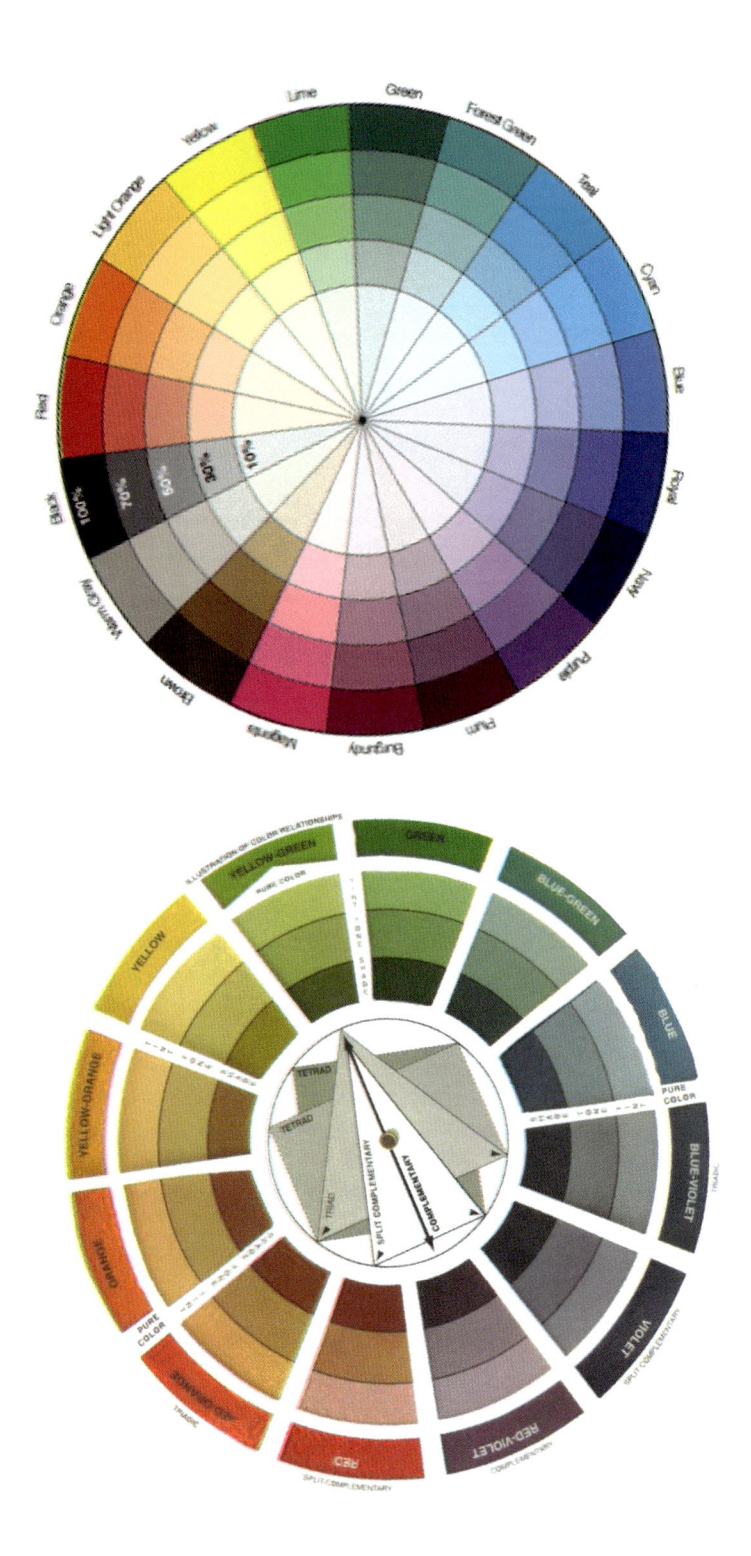

The examples we show here are just two color wheels from our collection. You can find color wheels in varying numbers and sizes. Choose one online at **www.colorwheelco.com**

How to Do a Color Analysis   16

Color Combinations

There are only six basic ways to combine color into successful and compatible clothing coordinates. Anything outside of these six ways creates an uncoordinated clash of colors.

Complementary

Colors that are opposite each other on the color wheel are considered to be complementary colors (example: red and green). Because of the high degree of contrast use these colors to stand out or make a statement. When stylists refer to contrasting colors they mean colors opposite each other on the color wheel.

Analogous

Analogous color schemes use colors that are next to each other on the color wheel. They usually match well and create serene and comfortable designs. Analogous colors are often referred to in styling as "monochromatic." In styling these neighboring colors are considered low-contrast.

Triad

A triadic color scheme uses colors that are evenly spaced around the color wheel. Triadic color harmonies tend to be vibrant, even if you use pale or unsaturated versions of hues. When styling triadic harmony successfully, colors should be carefully balanced - let one color dominate and use the two others for accent. In fashion triadic color combining is used to create coordinated outfits.

Split-Complementary

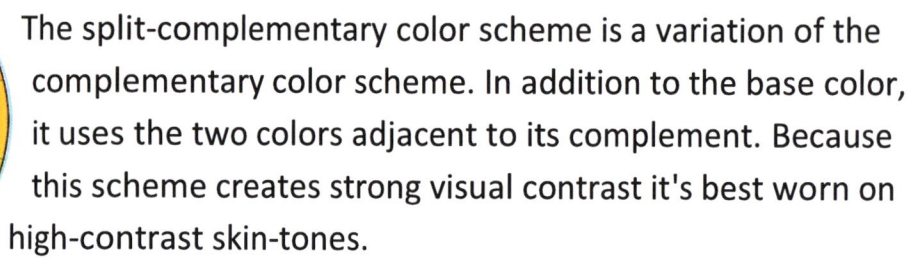

The split-complementary color scheme is a variation of the complementary color scheme. In addition to the base color, it uses the two colors adjacent to its complement. Because this scheme creates strong visual contrast it's best worn on high-contrast skin-tones.

Rectangle (tetradic)

The rectangle or tetradic color scheme uses four colors arranged into two complementary pairs. This rich color scheme offers plenty of possibilities for variation in styling. I elaborate on the use of rectangle color coordinating in Step 7. Here is an example of a tetradic scheme:

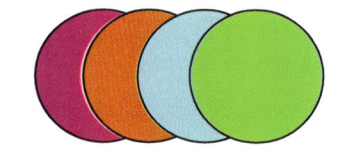

Square

The square color scheme is similar to the rectangle, but with all four colors spaced evenly around the color circle. Use four colors to create visually interesting and coordinated outfits. Square combining is often seen in menswear and interior design features.

The best way to learn how to mix and match colors using the coordination and combination rules above is to practice. You can also take a look at photos in magazines or at clothes hanging in a closet to contrast and compare the combinations that seem pleasing to your eye. Be sure to look for outfits that are compatible in one of six ways diagrammed above.

How to Do a Color Analysis   18

Color Theory

In the visual arts, color theory is a body of practical guidance to color mixing and to the visual impact of specific color combinations. Although color theory principles first appear in the writings of Leon Battista Alberti (c.1435) and the notebooks of Leonardo da Vinci (c.1490), a tradition of "colory theory" (as it was then referred to) really begins in the 18th century with a minor controversy over Isaac Newton's theory of color and the nature of so-called "primary colors."

Newton was the first to study and analyze the colors in a rainbow. He discovered that light, as viewed through our eyes, is refracted and that when external light hits a glass prism it has the capacity to create rainbow colors. Newton effectively proved that light alone was responsible for color. He diagrammed his observations on the refraction of colors formed by prisms into a circle of color and created the first color wheel. He identified colors opposite each other on this circle as complementary and their neighbors (secondary colors) as harmonious.

Color theory has long had the goal of predicting or specifying the color combinations that would work well together or appear harmonious. In the 20th century color theory attempted to link colors to particular emotional or subjective associations and color psychology was born: red is an arousing, sensual, feminine color; blue is a contemplative, serene, masculine color, and so on. This project has failed for several reasons, the most important being that cultural color associations play the dominant role in abstract color associations, and the impact of color in design is always affected by the context in which it is presented i.e., a red box has a different psychological association from a red dress.

However, many color trainers teach that when a specific color is worn for a specific occasion, celebration or situation, its impact can have negative and/ or positive consequences. An example of this would be if a red suit was worn to a funeral. The message sent by the wearer would be conflicting as red is a bright and powerful color whereas wearing a color such as black is sobering and more appropriate. Clearly, however, cultural norms play a significant role. For example, in much of Asia, white is the appropriate color for funerals.

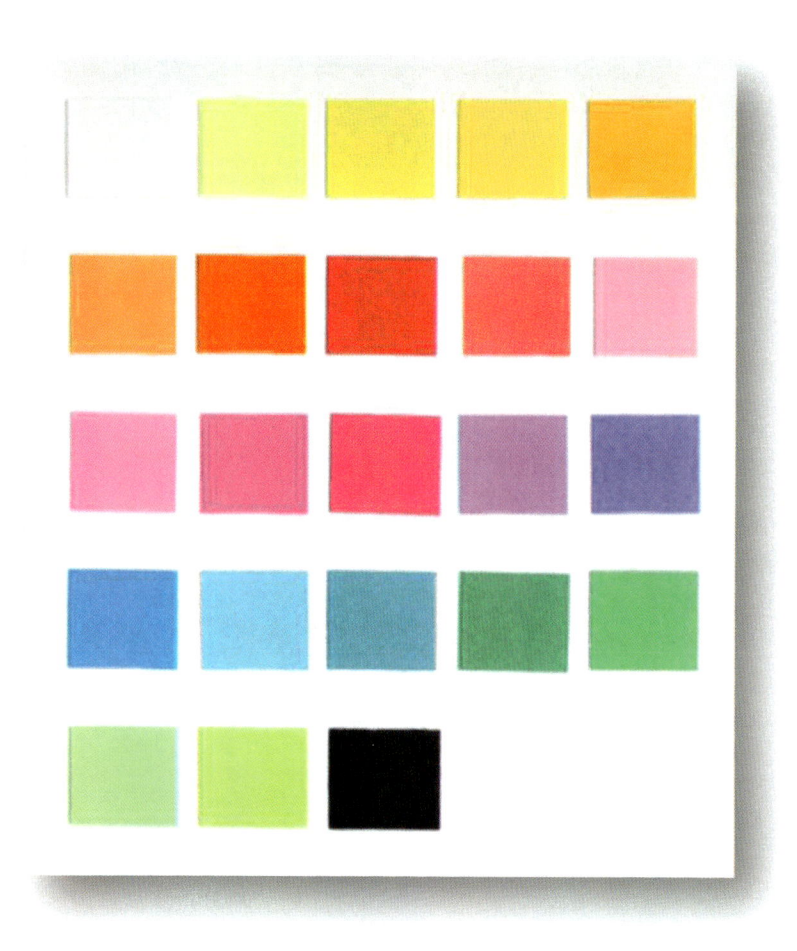

Example of a Color Scheme Using White Added to

Colors to Achieve 50% Saturation

The Color Wheel

A **color wheel** or **color circle** is an organization of color hues around a circle, showing relationships between colors considered to be primary colors, secondary colors, complementary colors, etc.

The color wheel has been adopted as a tool for defining these basic relationships. Some theorists and artists believe juxtapositions of complementary colors are said to produce a strong contrast or tension, because they annihilate each other when mixed; others believe the juxtapositions of complementary colors produce harmonious color interactions.

Colors adjacent to each other on the color wheel are called analogous colors. They tend to produce a single-hued or a dominant color experience. A split complementary color scheme employs a range of analogous hues, "split" from a basic key color, with the complementary color as contrast (red and orange). A triadic color scheme adopts any three colors approximately equidistant around the hue circle (blue, red, yellow).

Printers or photographers sometimes employ a duotone color scheme, generated as value gradations (such as shades of grey) and a single colored ink or color filter; painters sometimes refer to this effect as a monochromatic color scheme.

The color wheel harmonies have had limited practical application, simply because the impact of the color combinations can be very different, depending on the colors involved: the contrast between the complementary colors purple and green is much less impactful than the contrast between red and turquoise. Harmonies can suggest useful color combinations in fashion or interior design, but much also depends on the tastes, lifestyle and cultural norms of the consumer.

When color schemes have proven effective, it's often because of the fundamental contrast between warm and cool hues (hues opposing each other on the color wheel), the contrast of value with darks and lights, the contrast of saturated and unsaturated colors, or contrast of extension when one color is extended over a large area contrasting with another color extended over a very small area (for example placing a tiny black dot into a large field of white).

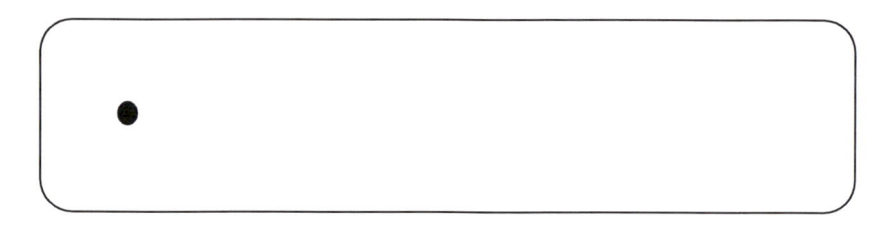

An Example of the Contrast of Extension

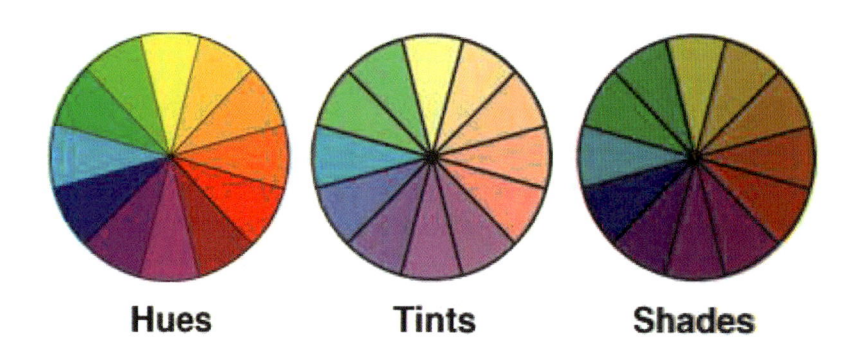

Hues **Tints** **Shades**

Chapter 2 - History of Color Analysis

Color analysis has been practiced in the United States for more than half a century, and it was in the early part of the 20th century that color consultants began utilizing a four-color system that corresponded with the four seasons of the year. Art educator Johannes Itten had already noted this natural correspondence of seasons and colors for decades. He stated, "I have never yet found anyone who failed to identify each or any season correctly. This demonstrates that above individual taste, there is a higher judgment in man, which, once appealed to, sustains what has general validity and overrules mere sentimental prejudice."

The concept of studying color in order to change and enhance the way a person looks was introduced in universities in the United States in the 1920's and 1930's, when home economics teachers passed along the principles of color from art studies to their students. Until that time, only artists were concerned with the study of colors and how their appearance could be manipulated and changed.

A few decades later, in California, U.S.A, Suzanne Caygill, a milliner and dress designer, created a color system that corresponded with the four seasons of the year, but for an unknown reason she reversed the names for the summer and winter color categories, and image consultants have continued with this erroneous classification ever since. In other words, she dubbed winter as a bright color category and summer as a muted color category.

It is important to know that a person's color season has nothing to do with the season of his or her birth or favorite season of the year. It is simply a way to name their skin's basic color tone (also known as undertone). Hair color may change over the years, while skin-tone may deepen with a tan, but in the color analysis system, an individual's basic color category remains the same.

It is also important to note that a person's coloring is established by the amount of melatonin in their layers of skin. Professional color analysis takes these factors into consideration when determining a person's skin-tone and color temperature while rendering an analysis of their appropriate undertone.

The first popular book on this system of color analysis, *Color Me Beautiful,* was published by Carole Jackson in 1980. Jackson also utilized the seasonal color system, but hers was less complicated than Caygill's. The book was an eighties pop-culture phenomenon.

Despite the development of other systems and more complex methods of categorization, the simple system in which colors are divided into four seasonal categories remains popular.

There is an enormous amount of research available regarding the science of skin color. When I started this book I discovered much useful information on Wikipedia (the free encyclopedia) and I have paraphrased here what I discovered. I strongly suggest you read up on this topic; it's interesting and can relate to successful color analysis.

Skin Coloring and Complexion

A person's complexion is a biological trait. The protein molecule known as melanin causes variation in tone. When melanin is present in higher quantities the skin is darker. Melanin is produced by cells called melanocytes. These melanocytes produce two types of melanin: pheomelanin (yellow/reddish hue) and eumelanin (dark brown skin and hair). The amount of melanin produced is controlled by genes in your skin cells and it is this genetic output that also controls how the skin colors from exposure to the sun. Through a process called *melanogenesis*, these cells produce melanin, which is a pigment found in the skin, eyes, and hair.

The allele gene found in melanin is responsible for the variations in skin tone across the world. Scientists know from research that one of these allele genes is responsible for 80% of all European and Asian skin tones and that the remaining 20% of humans have a mutation of an allele gene. It is a fact, however, that less than 100,000 years ago all human skin color was dark and as humans migrated north, out of Africa, to cooler climates, their skin adapted to the lowered levels of sun exposure.

A person's natural skin color has an impact on their reaction to exposure to the sun. The tone of human skin can vary from a dark brown to a nearly colorless pigmentation, which may appear reddish due to the blood in the skin. Europeans generally have lighter skin, hair, and eyes than any other group, although this is not always the case. Africans generally have darker skin, hair, and eyes, although this too is not universal.

Chart of Human Skin-Tones by Felix von Luschan 1854-1924

How to Do a Color Analysis 26

Application of Color to Consulting?

A recent ***Women's Wear Daily*** article mentioned a 2006 study done by L'Oreal Cosmetics which found that, based on exhaustive research, there are over 64 shades of skin tone in the world. "The realm of skin tones is vast, too, due to differences in undertone, unevenness of color...in Sweden, there are 21 of the 64 tonal classes in the fair end of the spectrum, while India, which, like Brazil, has had many ethnic migrations, has 40 of the 64 shades!"

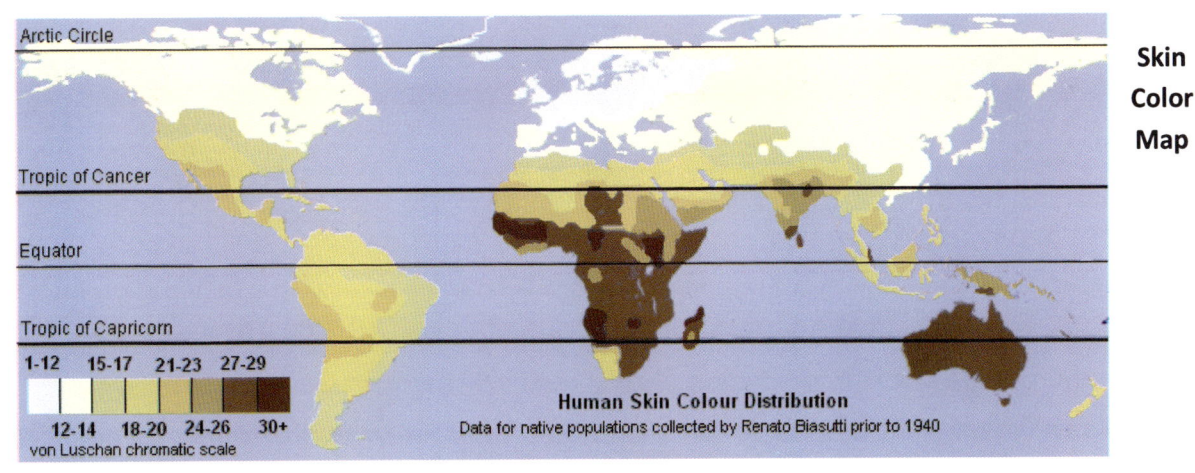

Skin Color Map

Composed By The Italian Geographer Renato Biasutti (Courtesy Wikipedia)

With statistics such as these it becomes clear that the work of color analysts is challenging. Being able to identify the underlying skin-tone of a client is at the heart of the work we do. By diagnosing correct skin-tones we guide clients toward the correct choices in makeup, hair color and clothing. Some color consultants also use color analysis systems in advising clients on the best colors for interiors in homes, cars and offices.

If you do a ***www.google.com*** search for **COLOR ANALYSIS** you will find hundreds of options for this service. I can't count the amount of different systems of color analysis being offered. I have seen variations on color analysis systems that range from 4, 8, 12 seasons (Spring, Summer etc.) to times of day (Sunset, Sunrise etc.) to gemstones (Topaz, Diamond etc.) to horoscope (reds for Gemini's, blues for Aries etc.) and even Feng Shui (as wood, water, earth). It's small wonder our clients get confused! Add to this mix the fact that many color consultants are untrained and provide incorrect advice to men and women and we are right back where we started - a bunch of people walking around in the wrong colors!

Color systems are not infallible; in fact, Carole Jackson herself has said that she believed her system to be imperfect. Color is not an exact science as so many of the options in choice depend on personal preference; however, there can be no doubt that skin-tones, because skin is composed of melanin (the primary determiner of skin color) can be measured as either cool or warm.

My system attempts to simplify this very confusing world of determining correct skin-tone. Condensing color analysis into just two temperatures of color allows an individual (and a consultant) many options in choice of color. Someone who is "warm" can wear all the warm based colors. Likewise a person who is cool can wear all cool colors successfully.

This does not mean that all warm or all cool colors will look the best and that's why I have added the second part of this system - 3D (three dimensions of hue, value and chroma). **2D/3D=EZ©** is a method that can be easily learned and effectively put into practice with the goal of providing CORRECT color analysis for clients. That's my goal - to make sure people are walking around in the right colors for them!

Consulting in 2D/3D

This system of color analysis takes into consideration a number of factors:

Skin Coloring – A person's skin color is the most important factor in determining which colors look best on them. Hair color and eye color, while equally important, play a less important role in determining a person's natural coloring. One's skin coloring is determined by the nature and proportion of the pigments contained in the skin cells just beneath the surface of the skin. Color consultants look for the color of the skins undertone to determine its temperature. During an analysis you will need to determine if your client is yellow based (warm) or blue based (cool) in temperature. Some clients might read olive based (this is also cool temperature).

Hair Coloring – colors can range from the lightest platinum blonde to the deepest jet black. Hair can have red, yellow, brown, black and even blue coloring. To get an accurate test of your clients natural hair color it helps if she has at least a half inch of growth at the roots.

Eye Coloring – The color of the eye determines its significance to inherent colors (best color choices) and even those flecks of color in the iris and whites of the eye will determine the best colors for a client to wear. For example - clients with rust flecks in the iris will look superb in rust colors worn close to the face.

Other factors to take into consideration when doing an analysis include skin texture (ruddy, freckled, spotty, luminous, creamy, smooth etc.) and contrast (low, medium or high), tooth color and whites of the eye. We will explore these factors later in the consultation process.

By using the **2D/3D=EZ**© system you can quickly determine your clients underlying skin-tone and advise her on the appropriate fashion colors to wear. You do not need to have my draping system in order to do these next ten steps. Although I do describe these steps on the assumption that you are using my draping system, you can easily use any existing drape system you already own.

2D drape system - I use three sets of drape categories: a set of cool, one set of warm and a neutral set that includes metal colors. Here is a short list:

Cool: black, white, burgundy, bright navy, cool taupe, Hunter green, charcoal gray, dark brown, orange red, vivid yellow, orange, emerald, kelly green, violet, ice pink, purple, dark blue, true red, deep purple, bright orange, electric blue.

Warm: ivory, pearl, amber, camel, mustard, warm beige, tobacco, gray green, olive green, coffee brown, coral salmon, apricot, moss green, terra-cotta, light brown, pumpkin, persimmon, golden orange, yellow orange, turquoise blue, teal, muted yellow green, burnt red, rusty brown.

Neutrals (include metal colors for jewelry testing): ivory, white, black, brown, gold, bronze, copper, pearl, red, orange, blue gray, green gray.

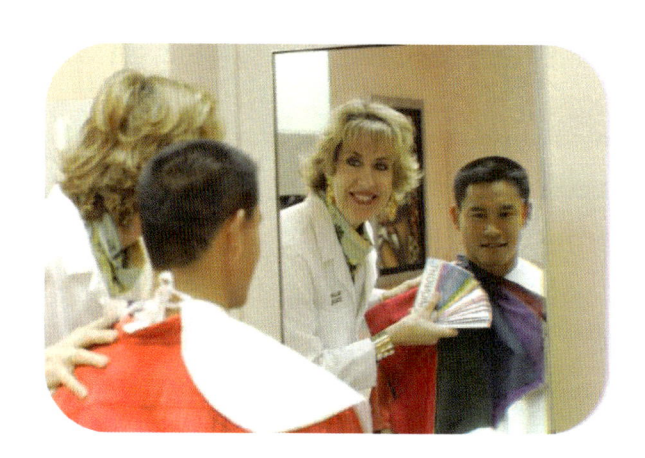

How to Do a Color Analysis

Chapter 3 - The Ten Steps

The Ten Steps to a Perfect Color Analysis

1) Prepare Your Tools, Supplies and Space

2) Client Interview & Color Questionnaire

3) Painting Skin Tone

4) Drape Tests

5) Hair Color Test

6) Analyze Skin Color Temperature

7) Color, Print and Texture Determination

8) Create Color Fan and Book

9) Makeup Consult

10) Offer Optional Services

Begin your color analysis practice by investing in high quality tools and supplies. In this chapter I detail the tools you will need, and where to get them. Have everything ready before you start working with clients.

Your work space needs to be clean, quiet and private. You will need natural lighting or natural light fluorescent bulbs if working indoors. Have all your forms ready for the client and have a clipboard for her to use. Make sure the room isn't too cold or hot and provide drinks.

Make sure that you have set up a private space with natural lighting for the color analysis. I use a swivel chair and place the client in front of a large mirror. I work from behind so I can reach the color drapes over her head and under her chin.

Be sure to advise your client prior to her session not to wear any makeup and to set her appointment with you when her colored hair has at least a half inch of grow-out at the roots. These two key points help you to make a correct analysis. You'll find a complete list of pre-appointment "to-do's" in the forms section of Chapter 5.

The first time you do a color analysis should not be on a paying client. Practice on friends and family first to iron out any areas you feel challenge you. Once you have mastered a consult with friends you will be ready to start consulting with clients by using these steps.

Remember - my system is very simple and should be easy for you to grasp. I detail quite a few tests you can do to be sure you are choosing one of only two correct underlying skin-tone temperatures.

The brochure on the next page is an example of an information sheet I send out to my clients prior to their appointment. You should create one of your own based on the steps you take to complete a color analysis session with clients. This helps prepare the client for what's to come.

COLOR ANAYLSIS SESSION

The colors we wear affect how others treat us; so, knowing the colors to wear for different occasions is an important component in your ability to affect and influence people. Knowing the psychology of color and how it affects you and those around you is the starting point of a custom color analysis at Gillian Armour Image Consulting. Your color analysis results are based on your skin pigmentation and your hair and eye coloring. We also look at your personal style, your personality and clothing favorites to determine your optimal color choices. We use a combination of professional color analysis systems to achieve your results. Gillian is a certified color analyst specializing in ethnic skin tones.

Components of a Custom Color Analysis:
- Color Chart Review
- Color Dimensions
- Color Harmony, Color Families
- Color Draping Test
- Color Psychology
- Hair Color Tests with Wigs and Hair Swatches
- Make Up Test
- Personal Pigmentation Painted
- Your Best Colors (dominant, power and signature)
- Determining Warm and Cool Based Colors
- Shopping for Your Colors
- Makeup Guide
- Personal Color Fan Creation

4 Step Action Plan:
- Interview, questionnaire
- Find Your Colors
- Creating a Custom Color Guide
- How to Choose Clothing When Shopping

Objectives of this session:
- Learn about color basics and theory
- Discover color psychology
- Dress with color confidence
- Realize your best hair color
- Wear color with confidence

What to Wear to Your Session:
- Something comfortable such as an oversized oxford shirt - preferably WHITE!
- No makeup
- Wear your hair back in a pony tail if it is long.

For the first few minutes of your session we will be discussing your needs. You will fill in a questionnaire that relates to your personal color preferences.

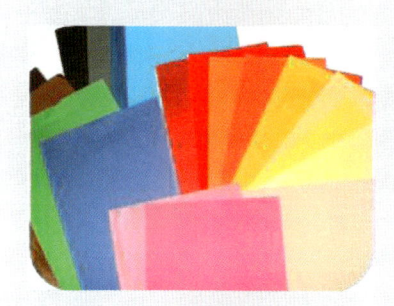

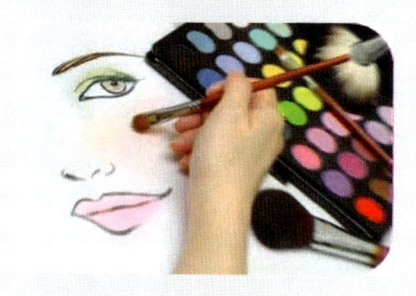

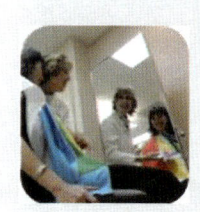

Please arrive on time for your appointment.
Do not wear any makeup and dress comfortably!

I look forward to seeing you soon, *Gillian Armour*

Pre-Appointment Instructions

Client Instruction List

Give your client this information sheet prior to her appointment with you.

In preparation of your initial **color consultation** with _____ please review the following.

1. Plan to spend 2 hours at your initial color analysis consultation.

2. Dress comfortably in loose fitted clothing. You will be sitting in a chair for most of the time.

3. Do not wear makeup and don't worry about how your face looks! We will be trying makeup on you during your session.

4. Do not wear nail polish. You will get a chance to see which colors look the best on you - including nail polishes.

5. Wear your hair down. If you color your hair schedule your visit with your consultant when you have 1/2 inch of root re-growth. This allows us to accurately see your natural hair color and helps us diagnose your underlying color temperature.

6. Bring a few pieces of clothing from your wardrobe in a color you are not sure suits you. We will review this at the end of your consultation.

7. This is **you** time so please don't bring your cell phone, kids or pets with you!

8. Don't buy any new clothes until after your color analysis. Likewise makeup, hair color and nail polish!

If you have any questions prior to your appointment please call_____.

Thank you. We look forward to seeing you soon.

Step One
Prepare Tools, Supplies and Space

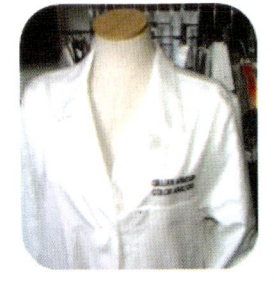

Lab Coat - I buy mine online at **www.labwear.com** and wear them when analyzing because it creates a color free background when the client is seated in front of me during the consult.

Bib - make sure you use clean bibs. I like the kind that tie or velcro around a clients neck so you can put them on and take them off easily. I also have a spare lab coat clients can wear if they feel more comfortable.

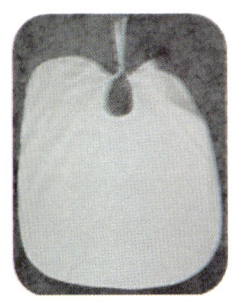

Embroidery Threads - these can be useful for illustrating colors in threads and fabric explanations to the client. I typically use them to show clients how color dyes work on fabric; how saturation of color occurs when dyes are applied to white.

Cool and Warm Lip Testers - a fast and effective way to test clients color temperature. I make these by painting lip shapes in coral and ice pink on plastic cards that measure 4" long by 2" wide. Hold these up to cover clients lips to determine cool or warm.

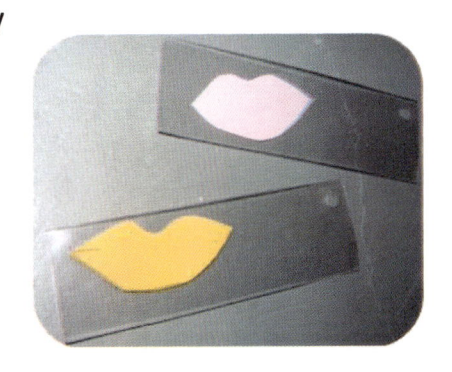

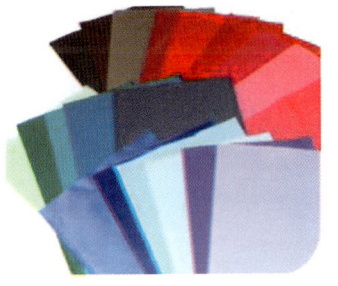

Drapes

You can easily make a set of your own drapes. Take a color wheel to the fabric store and match the colors on the wheel with fabric. I prefer 12" by 12" sizes but you can get drapes cut in any size. Be sure to mark fabric as it's cut - cool or warm.

How to Do a Color Analysis   37

Cool: black, white, burgundy, bright navy, cool taupe, Hunter green, charcoal gray, dark brown, orange red, vivid yellow, orange, emerald, kelly green, violet, ice pink, purple, dark blue, true red, deep purple, bright orange, electric blue.

Warm: ivory, pearl, amber, camel, mustard, ivory, warm beige, tobacco, gray green, olive green, coffee brown, coral salmon, apricot, moss green, terra-cotta, light brown, pumpkin, persimmon, golden orange, yellow orange, turquoise blue, teal, muted yellow green, burnt red, rusty brown.

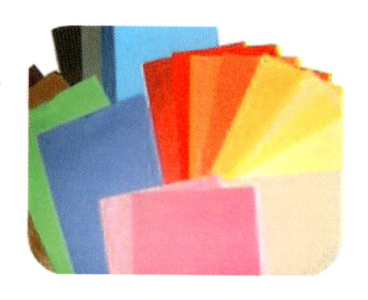

Neutrals: ivory, white, black, brown, gold, bronze, copper, pearl, red, orange, blue gray, green gray.

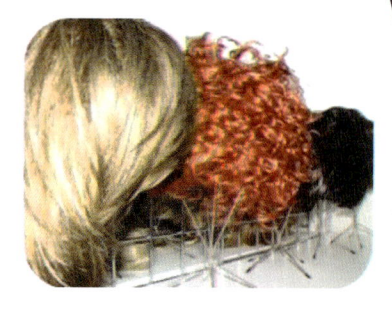

Wigs - selection of cool and warm hair. You will use these to affirm skin-tone temperature of cool or warm. Or use these for hairstyle consults if a client is thinking about changing her color or style.

Skin Color Testers - I have a set I painted myself and I also have a selection of charts that I've picked up from makeup counters over the years. You can also find paint cards at paint stores that will help you discover the client's skin-tone and to demonstrate makeup colors to her.

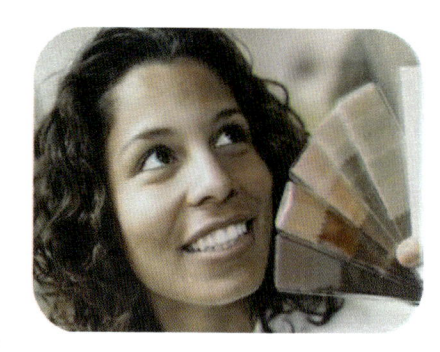

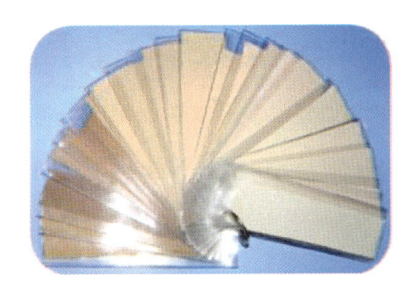

Make sure you test skin tones on natural, makeup free skin. If your client is already wearing makeup have her remove it. Be sure to have cleansers and cloth pads at the ready in case she needs to clean her face.

Hair Swatches to test natural hair color temperature - you can order these online at any wig site. Be sure to test close to her root growth in her center part at the crown or in the back of her head near the nape of the neck. If her hair has been recently dyed beyond its natural color you can ask her to point out from your swatches the closest match to her natural shade.

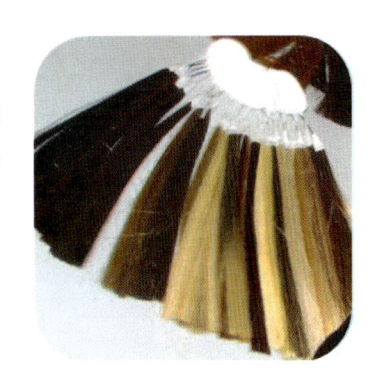

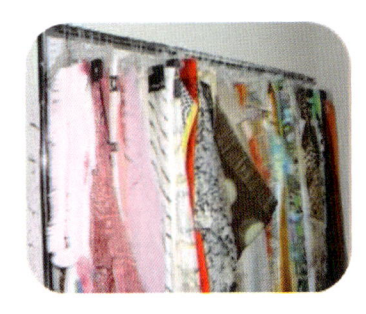

Collection Of Scarves - use scarves to test low, medium and high contrast. You will learn about contrast in Step 6. Organize your scarves separately by cool and warm.

Selection Of Jackets in both cool and warm colors.

These are great to have on hand as teaching tools for your client. You want her to be able to understand how her colors look on her before she leaves your studio. I also use jackets to teach clients how to wear colors that are not in her color fan. For example: if the client has tested warm and she says she has a cool jacket in her closet that she loves to wear, show her how to wear it so that her correct color is near her face.

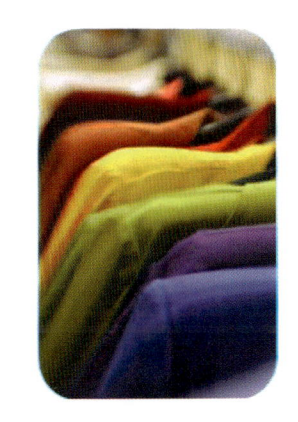

Take a scarf from your selection, and in her color temperature, one that coordinates with the jacket, and wrap it around her neck. Sampling colors close to the face in her temperature like this will show her that she can wear colors in another temperature. However, the best advice to give clients who have the wrong colors in their wardrobe is simply to tell them to get rid of them.

Box of Kleenex - just in case she needs to remove makeup or use to cover her face if she is taking off or trying on items of clothing.

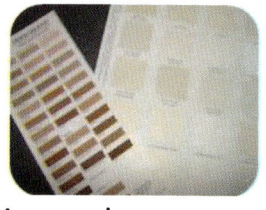

Makeup Selection - invest in a selection of makeup. You don't have to choose expensive make-up, drugstore varieties are fine. Ask your client beforehand if she has any skin sensitivities. If she does then use skin-sensitive makeup instead.

Makeup Applicators - visit any beauty supply store and stock up on mascara, sponge and eye makeup applicators. You want to assure your client that you are hygienic and use new applicators with each client.

Makeup Remover - have this on hand and be sure it is a skin-sensitive remover.

Mirror And Chair - A full length mirror is great, you can also use a half length mirror if you are working at a counter-top set-up. Find the system that feels most comfortable to you and is workable for a color consult. You do want to have counter space or a table nearby to hold all the tools you use during the session.

Be sure the chair is comfortable for the client and that her legs are not dangling in the air. I use a swivel chair that rises - similar to what you would find in a hair salon. That way I can raise or lower depending on the clients height.

Hand Mirror For Client - use a hand mirror with a handle so the client gets a close up view of how colors look on her.

Digital Camera - optional. Taking digital before and after photos is always fun for a client. She can see how she looks in both wrong and right colors. I also keep these as part of a client's file.

Selection of snacks and drinks - have these on hand to offer your client when she first comes through your door.

Step Two

Process client interview and forms

Welcome your client and have her fill out an application (I've provided a blank copy for you in the forms section) and offer her something to drink. Once she has filled out the client application proceed to this **Color Analysis Questionnaire**. Carefully note her answers as these will help you make a final determination of her underlying skin-tone temperature.

Start your analysis by asking the following questions. The answers you get will steer you toward a choice of warm or cool but the draping process in the color analysis itself will solidify a correct analysis of the client. I have identified **(C)** = cool and **(W)** = warm determinations for each answer. This will help you determine her underlying skin-tone. I have added notes to each of these questions to guide you toward making a proper diagnosis of your clients underlying skin-tone (temperature). Find your blank copy in Chapter 5.

COLOR ANALYSIS QUESTIONNAIRE

First Name_____ Last Name_____
Address: _____ City_____State____ Zip_____
Phone_____Email_____

1) Describe your facial skin coloring:

Pale and clear **(C)**
Fair with freckles **(C)**
Rosy (cheeks with a pink tinge) **(C)**
Ruddy (spots and colors) **(W)**
Tanned with golden highlights **(W)**
Dark with red cheeks **(C)**
Dark with golden cheeks **(W)**
Other:

2) Looking at your face in the mirror; how would you describe your overall skin tone?

Clear and Bright **(C)**
Soft and Muted **(W)**
Cool and Rosy **(C)**
Warm and Golden **(W)**
Light and Fair **(C)**
Deep and Rich **(W)**

3) When sun-tanning (with or without sunscreen) does your skin:

Burn easily **(W)**
Tan slowly - both
Tan fast **(C)**

4) What is your natural hair color?

Ash (dirty blond) **(W)**
Blond **(C)**
Gray **(C)**
Brown **(W)**
Black **(C)**
Red **(W)**
Auburn **(W)**
Other:

5) Describe the color or of your eyes:

Blue **(C)**
Green **(W)**
Hazel **(W)**
Brown **(W)**
Violet **(C)**
Other:

6) What color are the small flecks of color in your irises?

White **(C)**
Black **(C)**
Rust **(W)**
Yellow **(W)**
Deep Blue **(C)**

7) Go to your makeup bag, find your favorite lipstick color and write the name and brand here:

Lipstick names are sometimes a good indicator of underlying temperature- for example, a lipstick called 'icy pink' is probably cool, 'warm melon' is probably warm.

8) Which shade of lipstick do you prefer?

Pink **(C)**
Red **(C)**
Coral **(W)**
Beige **(W)**
Clear - both

9) What do you have more of in your jewelry box, silver or gold?

Clients who favor cooler colors will answer silver. Those who prefer warm colors will say gold.

10) Which colors would you wear if you could only choose three:

Coral, Buttermilk and Bronze **(W)**
Charcoal, Dusty Rose, Turquoise **(C)**
Ivory, Tomato Red, Turquoise **(W)**
Lemon Yellow, Fuchsia, Mint Green **(C)**

11) What ethnic background are you? Describe.

While it is not entirely necessary to know a person's ethnicity to determine their underlying skin-tone temperature, knowing it can lead you in the right direction. For instance, many Latin people (Italian or Spanish) have olive based skin tones. Usually olive skews toward a cool undertone.

12) What color is your car?

People usually choose possessions based on their favorite color. The answer to this question is not always an indicator of a cool or warm tone; some choose colors for practicality. You can also ask the client what her favorite color is. Her answer will also clue you in to her underlying skin-tone.

13) What is your FAVORITE color?

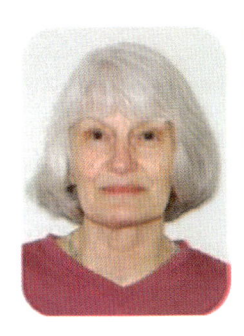

Next take a headshot photo. Find a white wall in your studio, preferably near natural light. If you don't have access to natural light you can get florescent and regular lightbulbs that mimic daylight. They are called full spectrum bulbs. Using your digital camera take a close up shot of the clients face. Be sure her hair is pulled off the face and that she isn't wearing any makeup.

Hint: if you want a true "before" picture don't coach her first. Photograph her candid, as she is. See example above. Usually photos like this make for dramatic before and after results. Once you have the candid shot then:

- Have client take off eyeglasses.
- Have client relax and stand against white wall.
- Stand 4 to 6 feet away from her and take a photo from a low angle.
- Take several head shots, both front and profile shots.
- If she wears glasses take a shot with her wearing them and then a shot with glasses off.

Remember that you will be editing the background of these photos later so definitely stick with a white background for your photo. When the client leaves and before your next session with her, edit the photos and file.

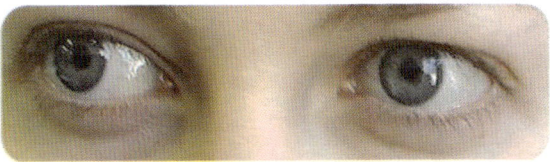

Eye Color/ Record - now lean in and take a long look at the iris in the clients eye. Make a note of the colors you find there. Look for tiny specks around the pupil and along the perimeter of the iris. These colors are known as "inherent" and are the colors your client can wear confidently. For example in this photo we can note that there is blue, deep green, light blue and pale yellow flecks in her iris's. She can wear these colors well.

Hair Color/ Record - in Step 5 you will test her hair against hair swatches. For your records just note her existing color. Ask her if this is natural or not and note the answer.

Three - Paint Skin Tone or Use Skin Testers

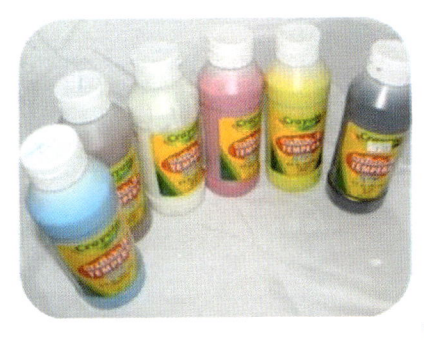

I use Crayola paint pigments for this exercise. The only colors you will need are magenta, cyan, yellow, black, brown and white. From just these colors you can create all the colors in the rainbow!

Begin with a blank piece of white paper. Using the white paint take a dime size dollop and put it on the paper. With your paint brush in hand begin adding tiny drops of magenta and blend.

To determine if your client has cool skin add a small drop of cyan (blue) paint to the white and magenta mix. You may need to add a small drop of black to darken this shade. Hold the color you have created next to her face and if the match needs to be lightened add white; darkened - add black. If this blue tone doesn't match it's now time to create a warm based skin tone.

Again, start with a white piece of paper, add the dollop of white paint, then the cyan. But this time add a tiny drop of yellow and see if the warm tone you create matches the client. You will have to play around to adjust the contrast values - adding white to lighten and brown to darken.

You can also match skin tone with complexion charts that you have collected and skip this painting process.

We have all heard skin described in many ways - ruddy, shiny, luminous etc. Be sure to determine your clients skin texture by testing various fabric drapes against her skin to see which ones harmonize the best. For example - someone with freckles all over her face will look exceptionally great in tweed fabrics with color flecks throughout. Someone with shiny skin (due to higher concentration of oils on the surface) looks great in shiny fabrics.

How to Do a Color Analysis

Four - Begin Draping Process

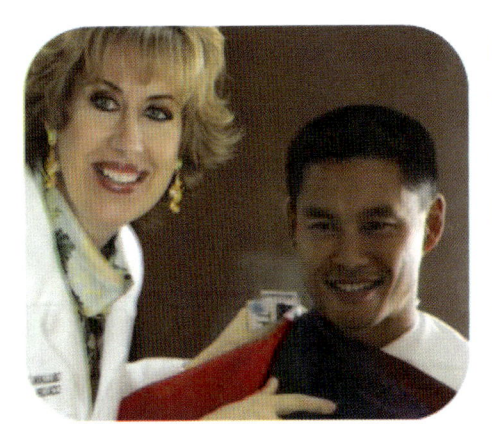

Now you begin the process of discovering colors that HARMONIZE, or blend, with the client's skin coloring. At this stage in the analysis you have probably determined client's skin-tone temperature but don't give away your answer yet. You do want to be certain of your choice. The drapes will determine your final answer!

For this step you will need:

A Set of Cool Colored Fabrics: black, white, burgundy, bright navy, cool taupe, Hunter green, charcoal gray, dark brown, orange red, vivid yellow, orange, emerald, kelly green, violet, ice pink, purple, dark blue, true red, deep purple, bright orange, electric blue.

A Set of Warm Colored Fabrics: ivory, pearl, amber, camel, mustard, warm beige, tobacco, gray green, olive green, coffee brown, coral salmon, apricot, moss green, terra-cotta, light brown, pumpkin, persimmon, golden orange, yellow orange, turquoise blue, teal, muted yellow green, burnt red, rusty brown.

A Set of Neutral Colored Fabrics: ivory, white, black, brown, gold, bronze, copper, pearl, red, orange, blue gray, green gray.

Fit one of the white bibs around the client's neck. Adjust the chair so you are not leaning down as you drape. With your drapes stacked on the counter or table next to you, hold one at a time close to the client's face.

Important - this is what I want you to look for: harmony. Allow me to explain in detail what should happen with your eye as you hold the colored drape of fabric under the chin of your client. This process happens very quickly once you get good at analysis so let me break it down some more until this comes naturally to you.

In the nanoseconds it takes for the brain to register if a color is attracting our attention the eyes have already done their work by fixing attention onto the color that is attracting them. If you put a color near the client's skin and watch where her eyes go this is an indication that you have chosen the correct color for her.

Let me explain a bit more so this concept is clear as several things happen all at once in this nanosecond:

1) the eye registers the color of the drape and seeks out a color that most dominates - if you put a white color drape on a warm skin-tone her natural facial color will drain away and the eye will attract to where dominance is.

2) the eye goes to where the dominant color has shifted - in our example the eye would travel to the white fabric itself because color has been drained from the face. White is not a color that throws light onto a warm face; in fact, it drains the facial color.

3) the eye now shifts back to the face to register the paleness of the skin, you will notice lines and skin imperfections because that is the only color that will remain on the facial skin drained of color.

4) you and the client will conclude that the color looks terrible.

Let me repeat this again because I want you to watch out where your client's eyes go when you put flattering and unflattering colored drapes below her chin:

If the eye travels to the fabric color first - this is the wrong color. If the eye travels to the face first, you've got the right color because the color is lighting up her features and harmonizing with her skin-tone. You will notice (and should point out to the client) that in the right colors her skin looks luminous, creamy and beautiful. THIS is the magic of color and how it can transform your clients if used properly.

Now you are ready to test her skin coloring with the drapes. Start with the set of neutral drapes. These drapes are a combination of cool and warm colors and should give you a clear indication of the ones that look the best. Progress through the neutrals making mental note of which colors looked the best.

Then move on to the cool drape set. Continue to hold each drape close to her face. You can make small talk as you go along but the object here is to see which of the colors harmonize with her facial coloring, which ones make her skin look terrific. You will start to notice a pattern once you are a few drapes in. The cool colors either will or won't look good. Continue to the end of the set and then start on the warm colored drapes. When you have finished going through all the drapes you should be able to make your determination of cool or warm temperature for your client. Make a note in her files.

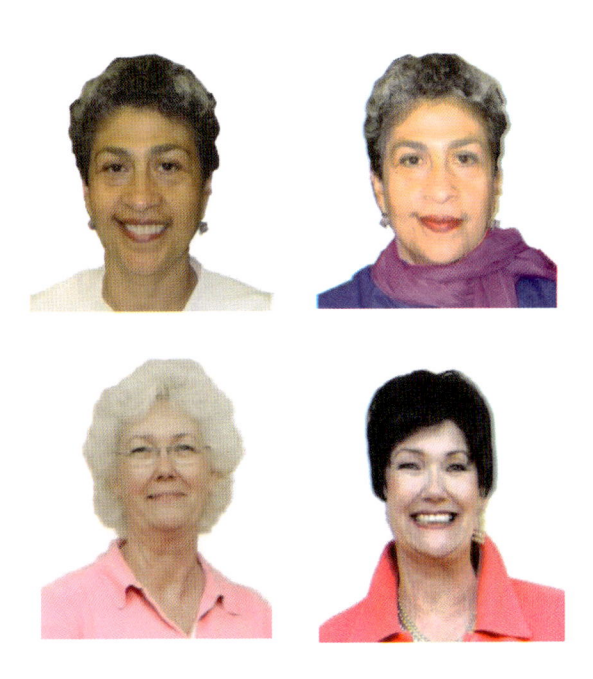

Before and After Color Analysis

Five - Test Hair Color with Hair Swatches

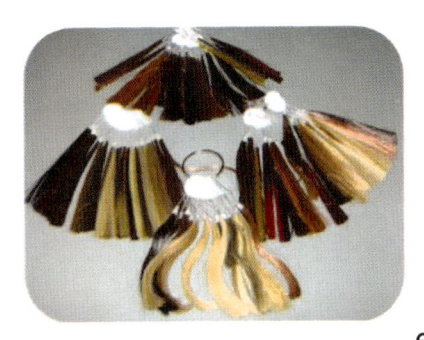

By now you have done five and even six tests to determine your client's underlying skin-tone temperature of cool or warm. Now it's time for one more test.

Hair color can be used to express personality, enhance facial features and improve mood. It can also be used to enhance eye color and to have psychological impact on the viewer. Because a person's hair is one of the first things we notice about them it's important to get the absolute correct color. Expect to spend some time with your client on this step of the consultation.

Chances are that her hair color is not appropriate for her skin coloring. Don't make an issue of it. As consultants we encourage, we don't criticize. When clients come to me I will observe if their hair color is either too cool or too warm so that once I get into Step 5 of the analysis I can start to show her the colors that are the perfect ones for her.

This step is crucial because hair color and style (and good makeup) can transform a woman. I also find it useful to do this step carefully as it encourages the client toward wearing her best hair color. You'd be surprised at how many of my clients come to me with the wrong hair color for their skin.

If you go online to any wig supplier you'll find hair swatches to buy. These swatches come in groupings of cool and warm shades. You can hold these up to your client's hair to match color and get a good reading of warm or cool.

Part your client's hair down the center part on the top of her head. Using your collection of hair swatches try to match one with her root color. When you find the exact or closest match make a note of it on the client form. She might also want to try on a few wigs to get an idea about style and color. I make this a teachable moment by having her try on both "correct" and "wrong" colors and styles.

Typically after a color consultation, and especially after trying on wigs, your client will begin to think about changing her color. She will want your educated opinion so study fashion magazines, online blogs or subscribe to newsfeeds about hairstyles to keep up with latest trends in hair. Make recommendations but stay away from determining what will look the best on her. Leave that up to her hairstylist. Here are a few **before** and **after** hair color and hairstyle looks! Much better!

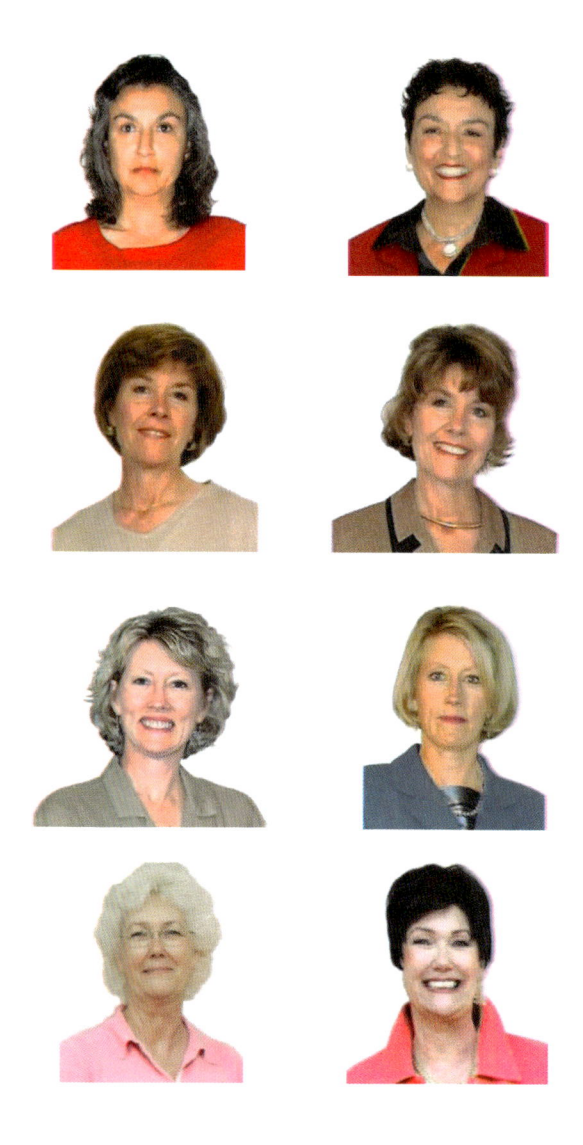

Six - Analyze Clients Coloring, Identify Contrast

Using notes you have taken and answers from the client's **Color Analysis Questionnaire** you can now determine if client is cool based or warm based.

Once you have diagnosed her you can begin to show her the color fans and all the colors she can wear. At this stage of the consult I begin talking about how she should use the color fan in her shopping, wardrobe editing, makeup purchases, etc.

Pull her fan from your stock and present it to her, explaining how the colors are arranged on the fan. Show her how to use the fan by holding the finger against clothing to get a match. Explain that when she is working with printed fabrics she should hold the entire color fan spread out to see if all the colors in the item harmonize with her fan.

Here is another exercise you can have her practice. Take a warm yellow jacket and a cool blue jacket (see our example on the next page). You should have one of each in your studio. Begin by showing her this easy way to differentiate cool colors from warm. Explain that when she is out shopping and doesn't have her fan with her the easiest way to double check if a color is cool or warm is to hold it up again a warm yellow or a cool blue item of clothing.

For example: she finds a cherry red top to buy. Her personal coloring temperature is cool. She can't quite tell by looking if the cherry red top is cool or warm. Show her what happens when you hold up a cherry red top against a warm yellow jacket. Ideally what happens is the red top now appears blue-ish because you can see the blue undertone in the red. Now show her what happens when you hold the cherry top against a cool blue jacket - it harmonizes. It goes with the cooler blue jacket because it has a cool undertone. Repeat the exercise again, only this time use a green top. Watch to see if the green harmonizes with the yellow jacket (which would make it a warm green) or with the blue jacket (cool green).

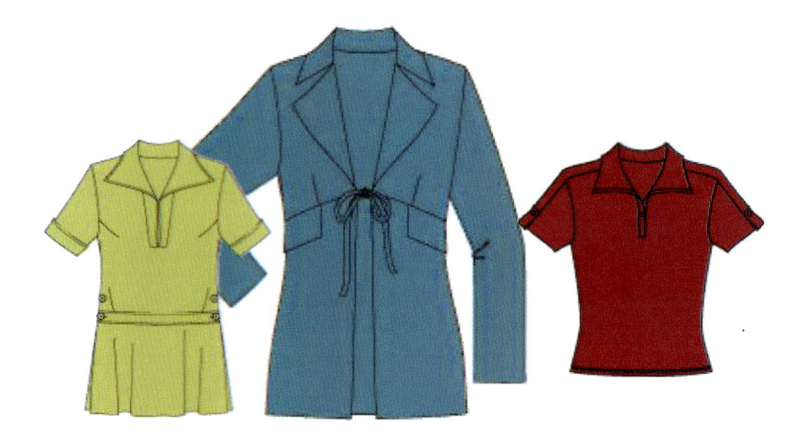

Which harmonizes with the blue based jacket? The green or the red top?

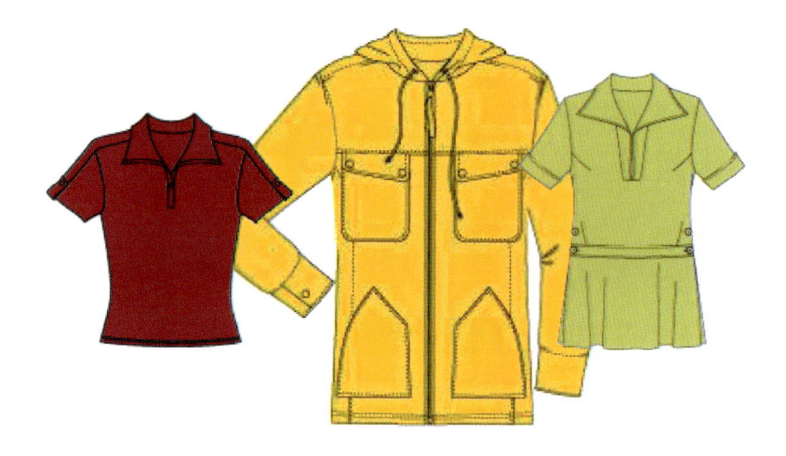

Which harmonizes with the yellow based jacket? The green or the red top?

Optional: Some color consultants will create a book for the client based on her best colors (inherent), power colors, colors to wear to lunch with colleagues etc. See "***The Power of Color in Your Wardrobe***" and "***Create a Personal Palette***" articles in the forms section and give to her.

Determine client's personal coloring contrast (low, medium, high):

Slight, visible or pronounced differences in color between eye, hair and skin will determine a person's personal coloring contrast. It's important to learn how to identify these differences in skin tone because a client's clothes should match this contrast in order to flatter her the most.

Low Contrast - identified as someone whose overall facial and hair coloring blends into one range of color values. Low contrast people have, for example, brown hair, brown eyes and brown skin. Or light skin, light eyes and light hair. There is no way to measure contrast so you will have to develop an eye for it. To determine if someone is low contrast notice if their teeth and the whites of their eye have little or no contrast with their skin tone. Next look to see if their hair color and skin color falls in with your low-contrast conclusion; if so, then the best prints for them to wear will be in the low contrast/ similar value range: deep red with red, pale ivory with white.

Medium Contrast skin tones will have more contrast between hair, eyes and skin and the color of their teeth and whites of their eyes will be brighter. Compared to a low-contrast skin-tone someone with medium contrast has more light behind their skin and a brighter smile. They look best in prints that are medium in contrast. Medium contrast color examples include pink with red, cream with brown.

High Contrast implies that there is a great degree of contrast between hair, eyes, skin, teeth and whites of eyes. A good example would be a woman with pale white skin, black hair and deep blue eyes - high contrast between all three components of facial contrasts.

On the following page you'll see examples of low, medium and high skin contrast.

Low Contrast	Medium Contrast	High Contrast
Slight to no contrast between hair, eye and skin color. Teeth are low contrast blending with skin tone.	Visible contrast between hair, eye and skin color. Teeth usually brighter in color than skin tone.	Pronounced contrast between hair, eye and skin color. Teeth match bright or light tone of skin.

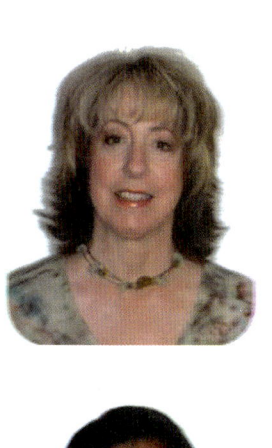

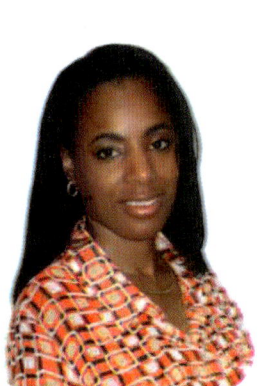

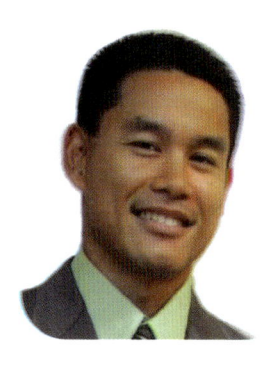

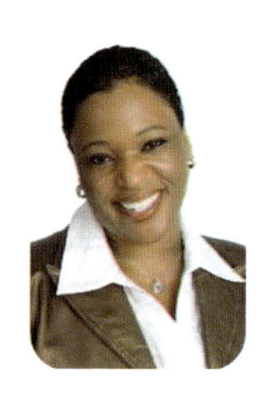

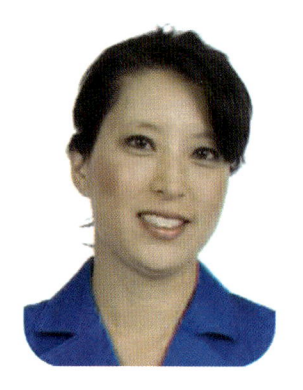

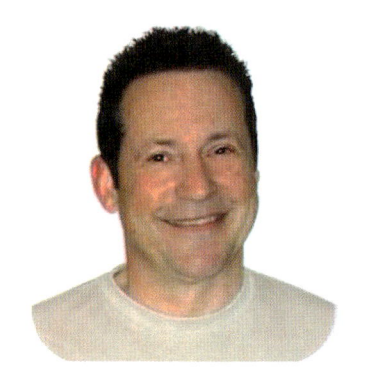

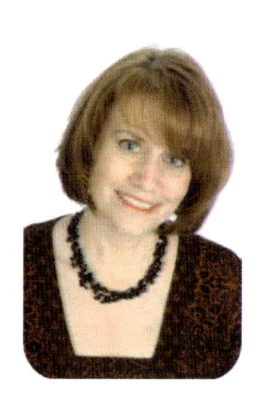

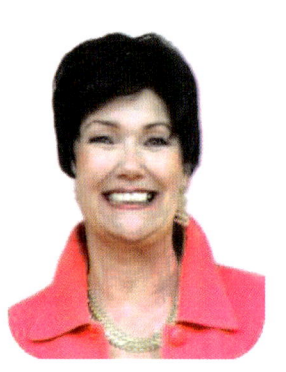

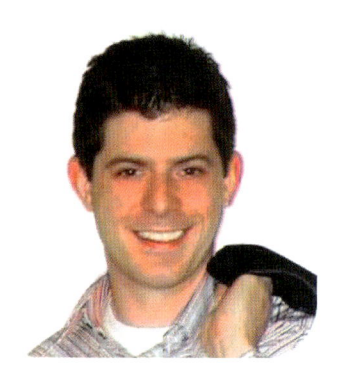

How to Do a Color Analysis

Seven - Demo Appropriate Colors, Prints, Textures and Contrasts

Based on your analysis of your clients skin, hair and eye contrast you have determined if she is low, medium or high contrast. At this stage in the analysis you will demo for her, using fabric swatches, scarves or jackets, how to choose correct contrast prints. These prints should match her individual contrast determined in Step 6. Be sure to have a selection of fabric swatches on hand (you can also use clothing) to demonstrate your points to the client.

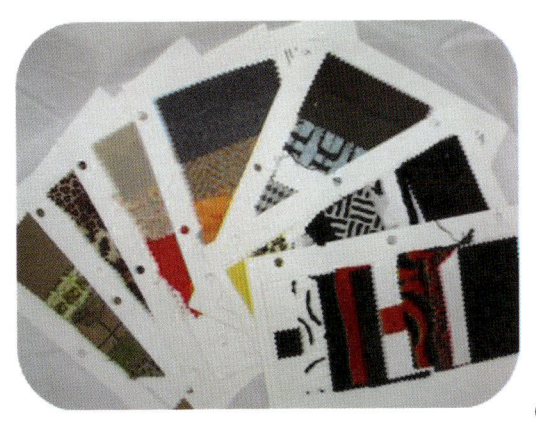

Here is an example of contrasting print fabric swatches I use for demonstration purposes. Yours should consist of low contrast (pale pink with hot pink), medium contrast (pink with red) and high contrast (pink with black) samples. My swatches include examples of prints, textures and fabrics. Create your own easily by visiting a fabric store to purchase inexpensive pieces of fabric leftovers.

How to Mix and Match Colors and Patterns Successfully

Understanding how to mix colors is essential to creating an effect that is both pleasing and harmonious. To get ideas, look for color schemes you find attractive, not only in fashion spreads and ads in magazines, but in fine arts, paintings, and nature.

Learning to combine various shades correctly, and avoid those that don't mix well, is part of using color to its fullest power. Black, for instance, looks great with shocking pink, peach, lemon yellow, or pale blue. Shades of beige look wonderful with red or peach. Navy is elegant accented with red or pink. Wearing a red wrap with a navy suit and classic white shirt, adds an uplifting color, as does wearing a shocking pink scarf across a black suit. The following color charts are for you to practice with. Try to match colors from the same cool and warm families to get coordinated outfits.

Cool Color Fan

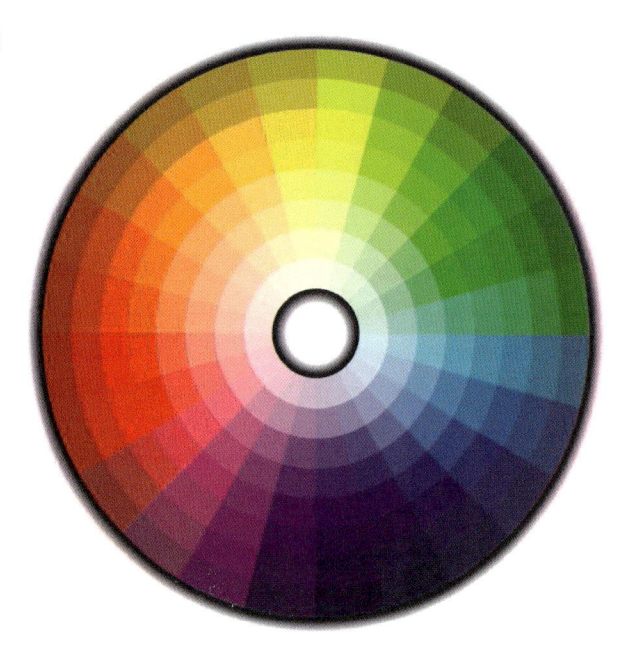

Warm Color Fan

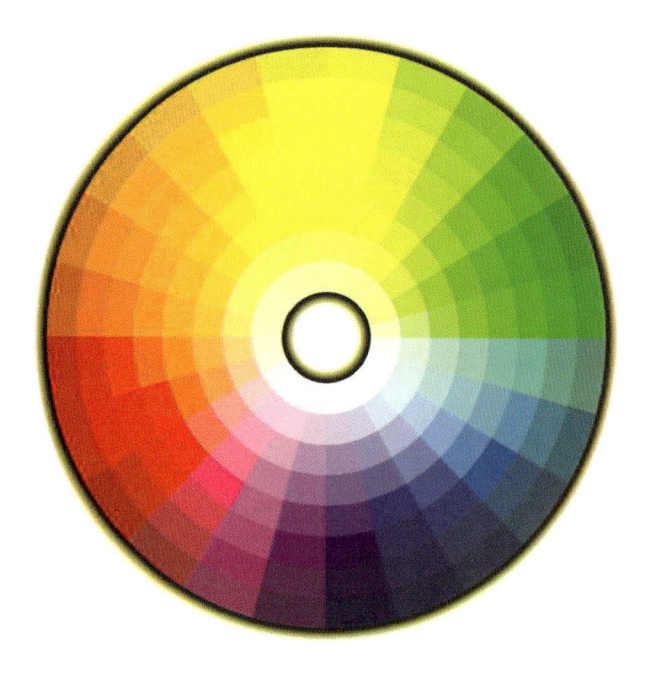

One of the best visual examples of mixing and matching happens in nature. The natural world brims with examples of colors that work well together. Take a cue from this world and pick up a few pointers for your own color coordinating skills.

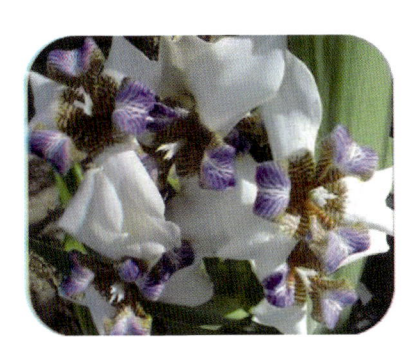

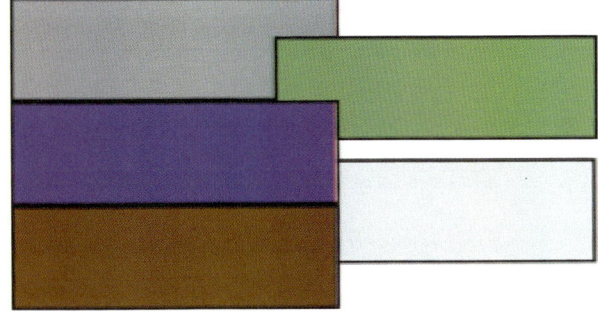

Here is an example that can help us determine colors that go together. In the photograph of irises above there are many colors. I have separated out the most DOMINANT of these colors into the boxes on the right. With these five colors you have the foundation of a well-coordinated outfit.

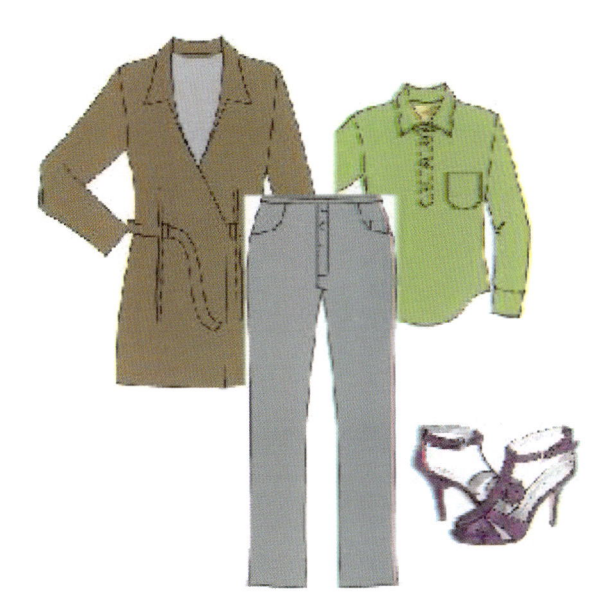

Let's break down the colors we pulled out of the picture of the irises. Notice these colors aren't too bright, too dark, too soft or too hard. Each one of them is in the medium range of the color wheel - we can say 50% saturated with white (adding white lightens them from their original color). Also notice they each harmonize, "go" with each other; they are not opposite to each other on the color wheel but instead are close and friendly neighbors who can get along.

How to Do a Color Analysis

In this example we have used four colors to create an outfit. If a fifth color were added it would have to be in a tiny quantity (a pin on a lapel) to avoid looking overdone.

√ Each item is in the same range of color saturation

√ Each one is a close neighbor

√ Up to four different colors can be used to create an outfit. Any more and you risk looking over-the-top!

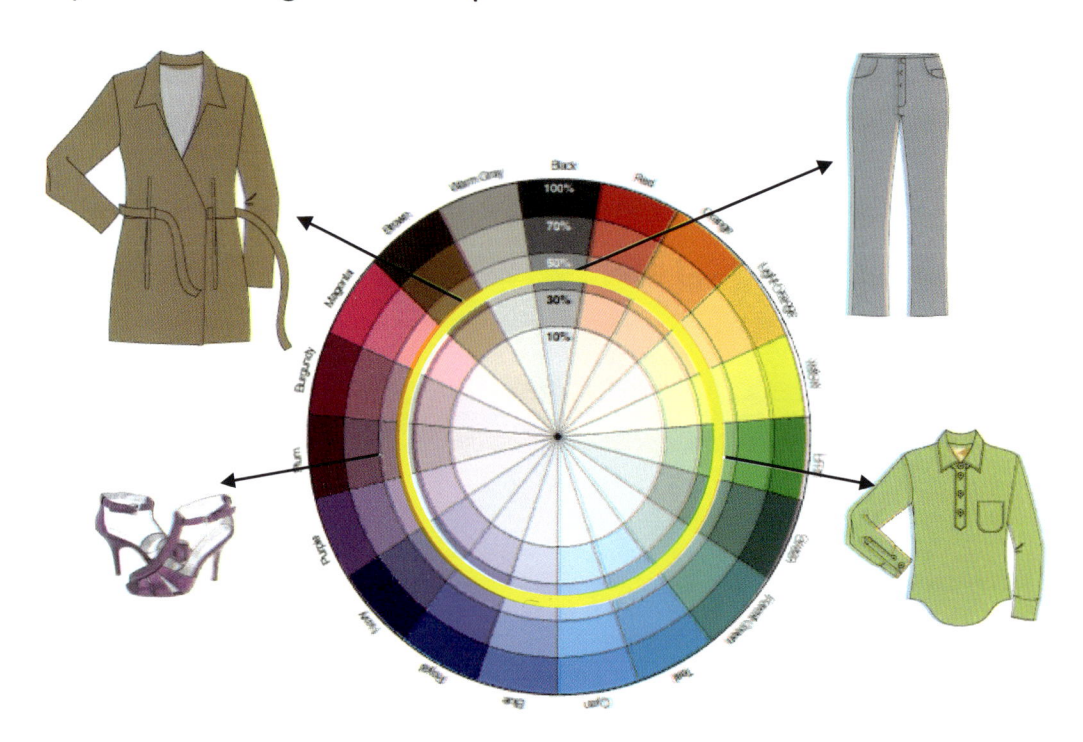

Taking our analysis of this outfit one step further let's look at the primary and secondary silhouettes of clothing. Our primary (basic) pieces include the jacket and the pants. Our secondary (accent) items are the blouse and shoes. Here is the rule for this outfit: primary items are neighbors, secondary items live across the way from each other.

These swatches represent clothing fabrics and textures. The three swatches and accessory swatch make up one complete outfit. These colors are known as a range and are in harmony within the color families they represent.

How to Do a Color Analysis   62

When you pull outfits together based on these four rules of coordination you can't go wrong.

- **Basic** - the most dominant item of clothing, usually what's on top.
- **Accent** - the color that ties together the basic clothing item with the neutral.
- **Neutral** - typically the final item of clothing, usually a basic pant, skirt or short.
- **Accessory** - the color of an item that ties the outfit together. Scarf, jewel, handbag, shoe etc.

BASIC

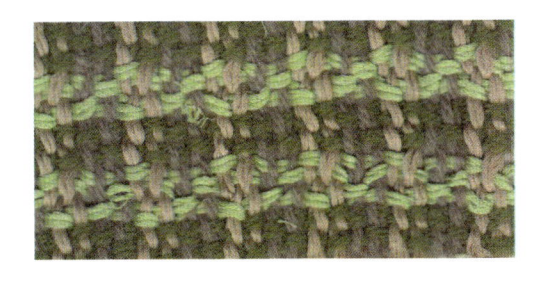

NEUTRAL

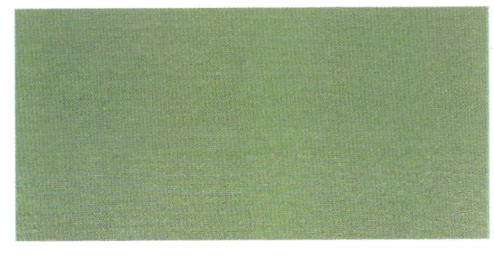

ACCENT

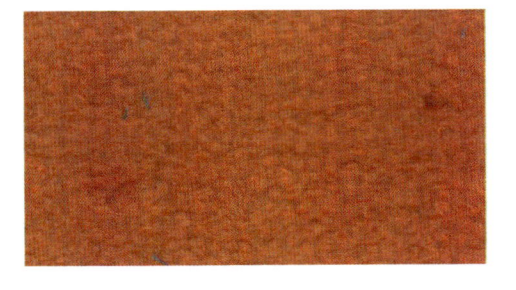

ACCESSORY

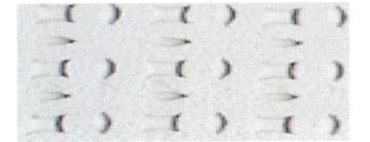

How to Do a Color Analysis

Universal Colors

There are some colors from both the warm and cool sides of the color wheel that can be considered universal. These colors look good on most skin tones and are best used when the choice of clothing worn has to be the same for everyone; situations such as uniforms or bridesmaids' dresses, grooms' bow ties etc.

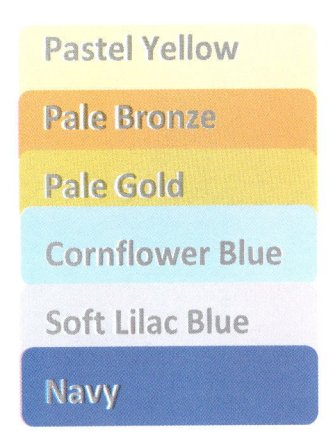

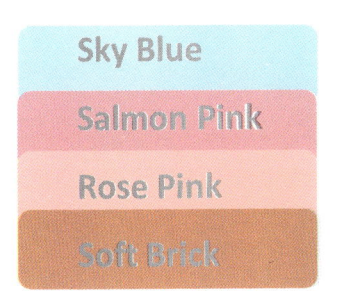

- Pastel Yellow
- Pale Bronze
- Pale Gold
- Cornflower Blue
- Soft Lilac Blue
- Navy

- Sky Blue
- Salmon Pink
- Rose Pink
- Soft Brick

Universal Neutral Colors

Black, white, grey, and navy (cool colors) can be worn by everyone as a basic, however, it's best to use an accessory such as a scarf, or shawl, nearer to the face if a person has a warm underlying skin-tone. As a color analyst you should add these neutrals into your color fan palettes or, if you are using ready-made color fans from a reputable color consultant, these neutrals will be included in the fans.

Coordination Success

Additional key points to remember when coordinating clothing – be sure to include fabric, texture, print, style and silhouette. Each of these elements make up a successful outfit and each one must be accurately coordinated. Here are the guidelines for successful coordinating: (learn more about these concepts in my book **"How to Do an Image Consult"**)

Fabric - textiles play an important role in the clothing styles of today. Natural fabrics have made way for synthetics as the easier choice for wear and care.

Texture - fabric textures (and prints) come in different weights: small, medium and large. Do not overpower a client's body type with the wrong texture of fabric. If she is small boned she should not wear large textures such as nubby bouclé or thick corduroy.

Print - big prints and busy visual action can make a large person look larger; likewise a small print diminishes a petite person.

Style - can be learned and reflects the taste level of the wearer. Do not cookie-cutter the fashion choices for your client. Learn how to be creative with your styling and coordinating to better teach your clients how to do this.

Silhouette - finally, the line and proportion of clothing create the silhouette (shape) of the body. You can create an hourglass shape even if your client's figure isn't one. Clothing comes in so many styles and silhouettes that creating a long, lean and curvy shape is easy.

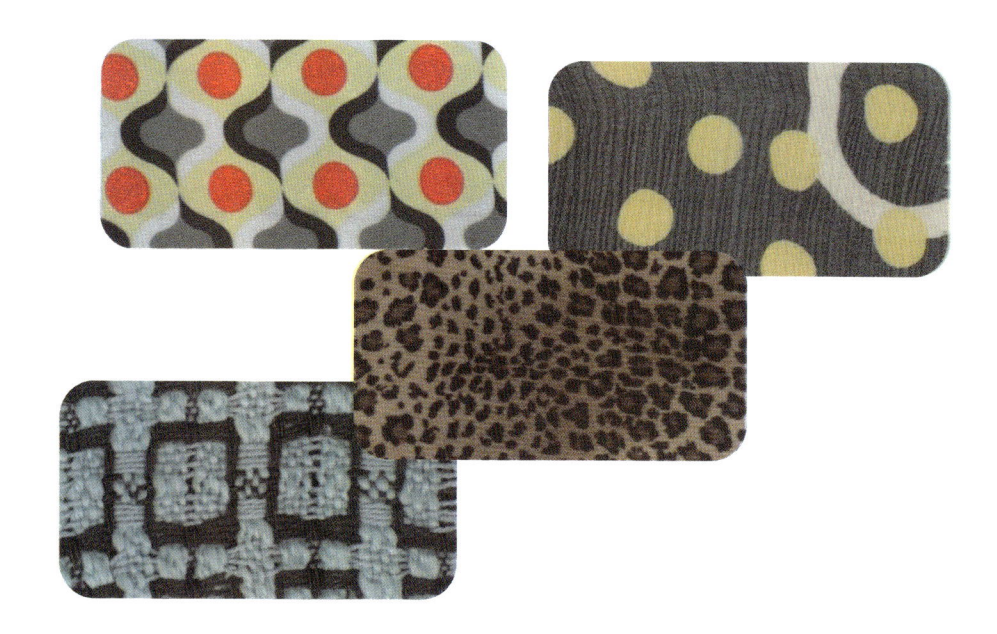

Practice Session

Now that you know how to coordinate colors, you need practice. Get your hands on a recent fashion magazine.

First - Cut out photos of styles to coordinate. If the photo you view is already coordinated just cut out one item – main, basic, accent or accessory and collage your own coordinated outfit.

Second - Once collaged determine the color relationships of all the pieces in the coordinated outfit. Are they all within the same color family? Is there one color piece that is from the opposite side of this color family? When deciding how to pull a coordinated outfit together you will need to consider these points and more.

Third - Keep making collages. These will become the basis of your portfolio and an invaluable tool to use when presenting ideas to clients.

I have found a great resource for teaching clients how to mix and match; pay a visit to ***www.polyvore.com*** and begin learning how to coordinate clothing styles, silhouettes and color.

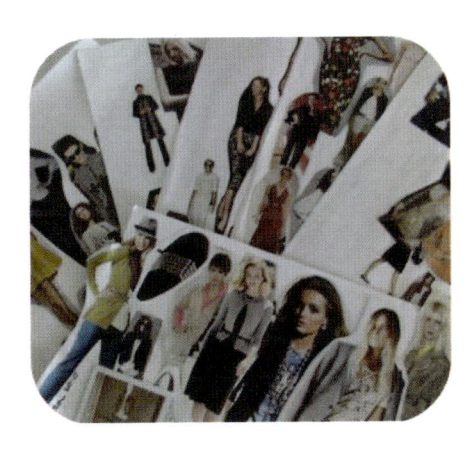

Collage or Story Board Example

Color Images

After I have completed a color analysis of a client, I will create a color book for her. This book is separate from her color fan and includes information relevant to the understanding of color. I will fill it with interesting articles, illustrations and will also collage multiple outfits for my clients to wear using jpeg images I have created.

These are available on my website (www.fashionimageinstitute.com) as **Mix and Match Jpeg Image System**. Here is a sample of a page I put together recently for a warm temperature client.

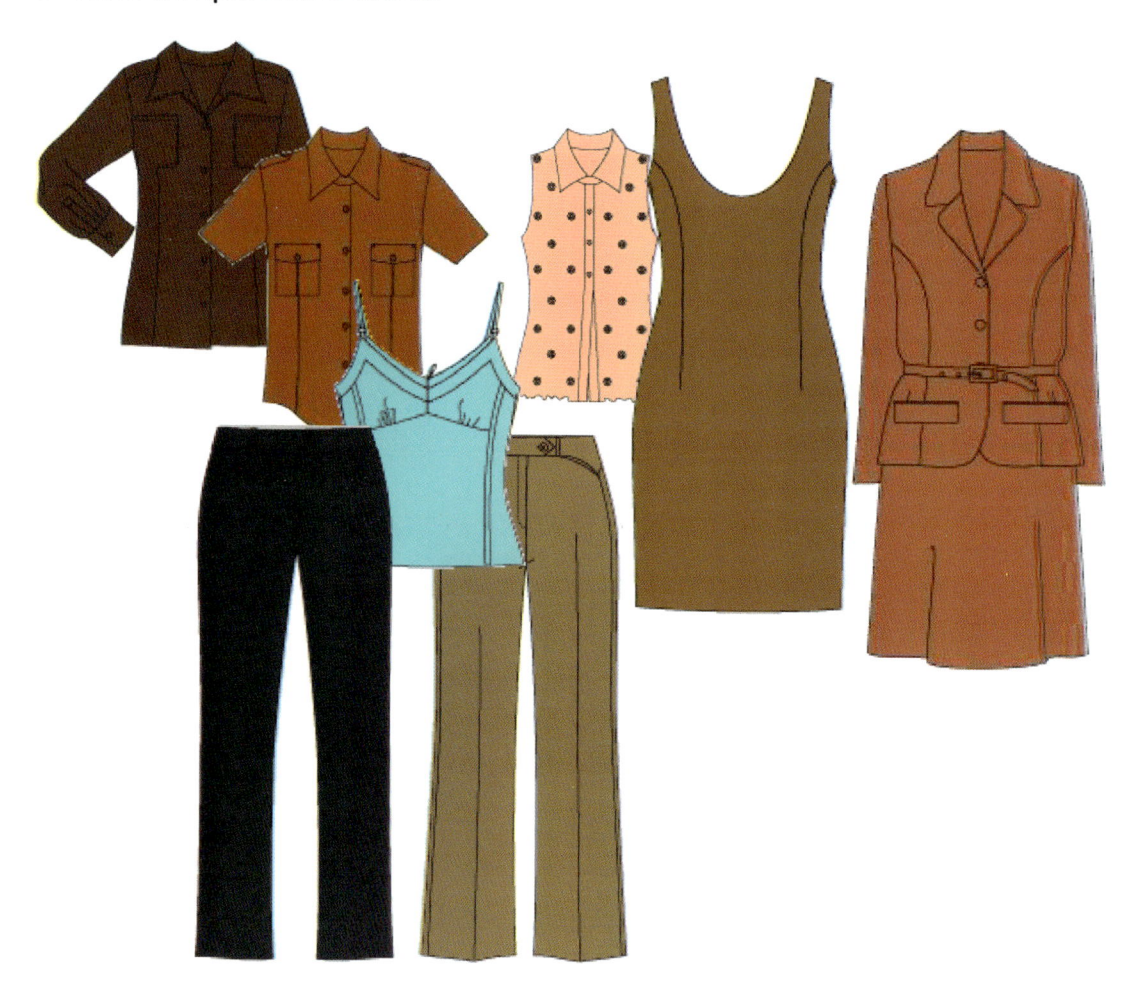

How to Do a Color Analysis   68

Eight - Create Clients Color Fan/ Book

A color fan is a selection of fabric or paint examples in a range of colors that match your client's underlying skin-tone temperature. In order to custom create your client's final fan you will need to either have fabric stock on hand or buy color swatches from an existing color consultant.

While some color consultants will sell their color fans, most will not sell to you until you have trained in how to facilitate an analysis following their methods. We do stock both cool and warm color fans. You will find them on our website.

Ideally the fan should hold a minimum of 48 colors and include the metal and neutral colors. Your clients will need this range of colors in order to identify correct clothing when they shop.

Your clients will benefit from articles that explain more about the world of color (I have supplied you with a few in Chapter 5). Write your own, or find a book you like and recommend it to clients. If you come across an interesting article send it to them.

When you review the color fan with your client explain that this is a powerful tool she can use to edit her existing wardrobe to cull unsuitable colors. The color fan is also great to use when shopping for coordinated shoes, accessories, jewels and even makeup colors.

Note: if you are creating your own fans from color fabric swatches and preparing a color book for your client, it's best to do this when the client is not around. Set up a separate appointment with her after you have tested the drapes on her to review all her color choices.

Customized Fabric Swatch Books for Clients

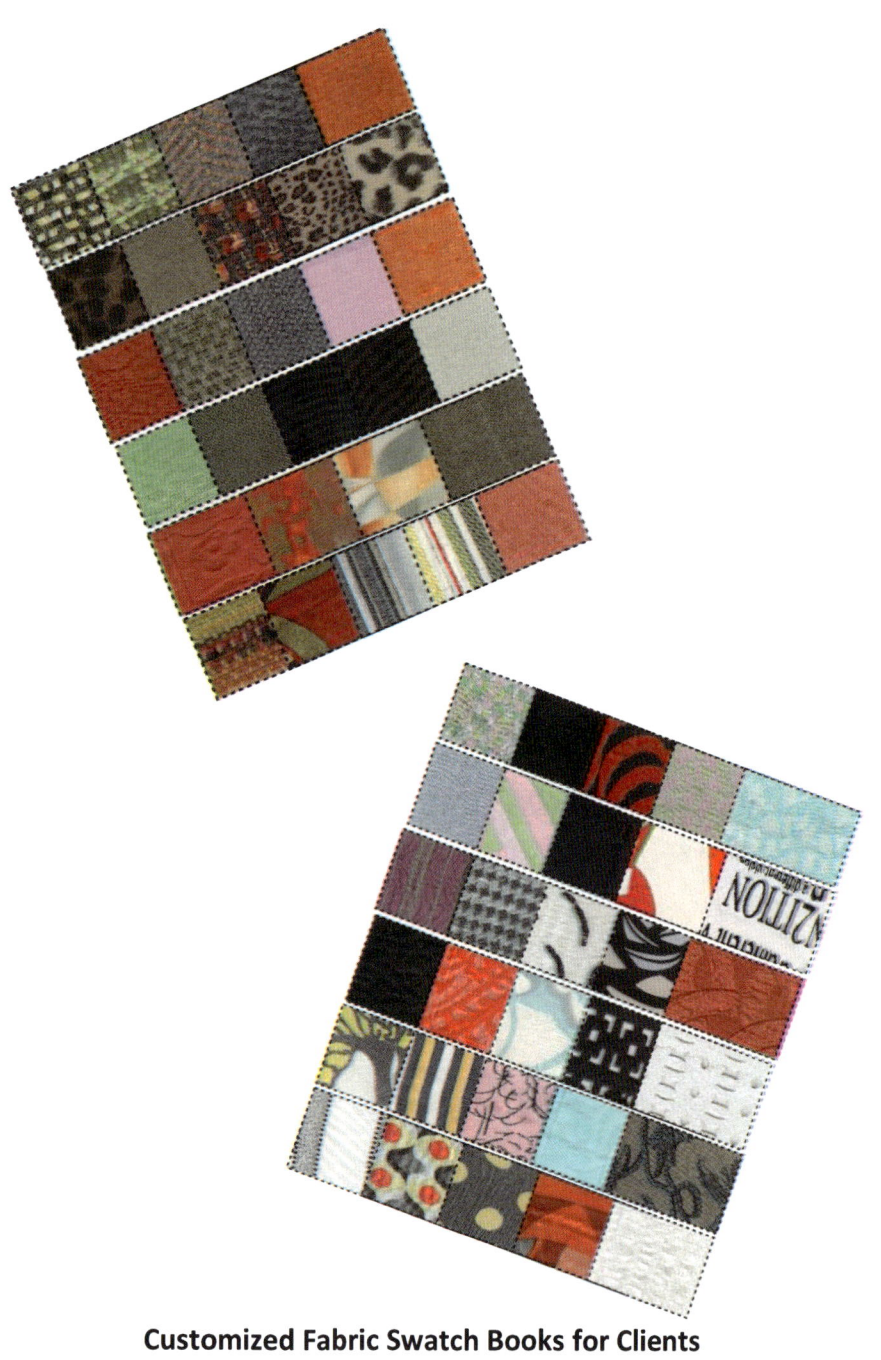

Nine - Detail Appropriate Makeup

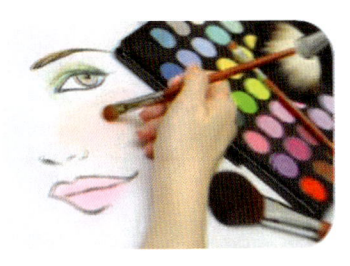

Once you have diagnosed your client's underlying skin-tone it is easy to recommend makeup colors that will suit her. You can use her color fan or you can walk her through a makeup application session. Be sure to have a selection of makeup products on hand if you are doing a makeup session.

The makeup chart listed here is just a guide. Unless you have makeup training it's best to leave makeup application to the pros. Take your client to the makeup counter of a nearby department store and have a makeup artist apply correct colors based on your analysis of her skin-tone.

Makeup affords women a simple, effective and inexpensive way to dramatically enhance or change their appearance. The right makeup color and application can make us positively glow, while the wrong makeup color or application can ruin an otherwise perfect look. If you are skilled in makeup application it's always fun to show your client her best and worst colors. The following exercise should be done in the spirit of teaching.

With client seated in front of the mirror, and holding a hand mirror, demonstrate with eye makeup colors the best colors for her on one eye and the worst colors on the other eye. Point out that you have used her inherent colors (all the colors you found in her irises in Step 2) on the "right" side. She will be very surprised to see how the "wrong" side looks in comparison. For the "wrong" side use makeup colors from the opposing temperature palette (warm if cool, cool if warm).

I also take this time to talk about nail polish as well. As in makeup, there are warm and cool colors in polish. Be sure to choose the right one for her.

To help you learn more about makeup application and techniques I have written a professional guide "Face Design and Makeup." *(See resources.)*

COLORING	MAKEUP FAMILY
Dark Hair/ Olive Skin	Warm Brown
Brunette/ Warm Skin	Warm Peach
Brunette/ Cool Skin	Soft Peach
Dark Hair/ Warm Skin	Rosy Brown
Dark Hair/ Cool Skin	Cool Rose
Blonde Hair/ Warm Skin	Tawny Pink
Blond Hair/ Cool Skin	Baby Pink

Color Chart from "Face Design and Makeup" by Gillian Armour

How to Do a Color Analysis

Step Ten - Add on Services

Shopping - This final step is a separate consultation with your client. If you do personal shopping trips then you already know you need to have your client's color file with you when you shop. Some consultants keep a copy of the client's actual color fan and will shop for, or with her based on this fan.

Teaching your client how to shop on her own with her color fan should first be taught by using scarves, jackets and fabric samples as we have already shown you. Take her shopping to show her how to use the fan. This is a great way to introduce her to the challenges of shopping by color!

Closet Editing - her color fan is an ideal tool to use when doing a closet audit. Again, you can create a separate session (and charge for it) to edit her closet. Pull items that are not in her color fan and get rid of them. Using the color fan is a great way to pare down an overstuffed closet.

Makeup Application and Shopping - don't combine a makeup shopping trip with a clothing one. Makeup application takes a lot of time and you don't want to overwhelm a client. Pay a visit to the makeup counter with your client and put her into the hands of a makeup professional.

Accessory Editing and Organizing - the color fan can be used to edit scarf, handbag and jewelry collections. I once had a client insist that her shoes be edited and only the correct colors be left in her wardrobe!

Office Interiors - since color affects our mood it helps to have our best colors surrounding us in our work environment. Use the color fan to coordinate interior decorations and wall paints. Help your clients create personal spaces that harmonize and make them feel good!

Color Trend Reports - I don't charge clients for my color trend reports. I go to *www.pantone.com* each season and get the full color trend report of the season. I then synthesize the information into a one-sheet page and email it out to clients. This report gives my clients ideas for the coming season and details colors that will be in fashion. I also create a spreadsheet with trend colors to show my clients how to mix and match clothing. Here is an example of this coordinates report.

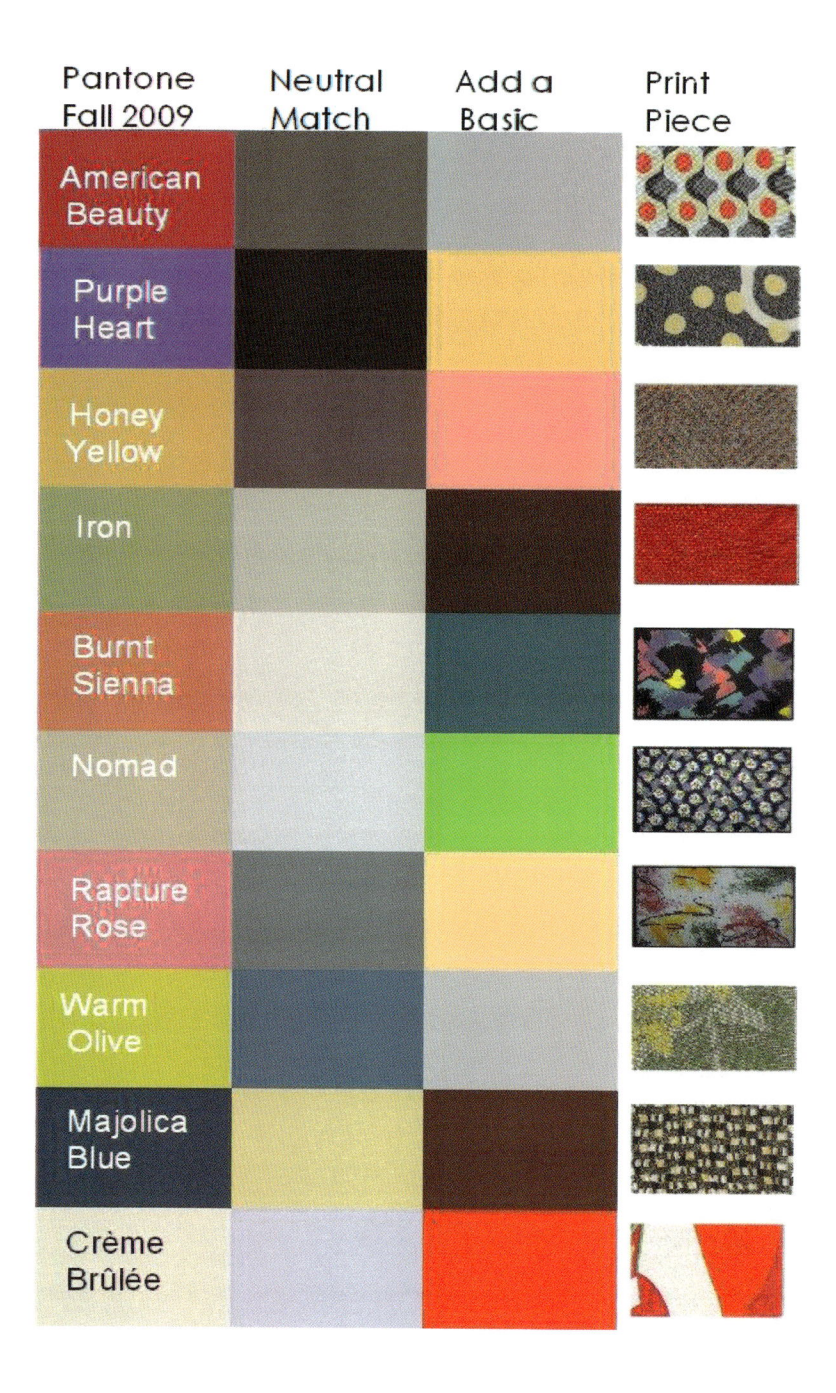

Pantone Fall 2009	Neutral Match	Add a Basic	Print Piece
American Beauty			
Purple Heart			
Honey Yellow			
Iron			
Burnt Sienna			
Nomad			
Rapture Rose			
Warm Olive			
Majolica Blue			
Crème Brûlée			

How to Do a Color Analysis   74

CH 4 Marketing Your Business

At the start of your business you will rely on networking to get the word out about your services as a Color Consultant. That means every person you meet and each project you work on should serve as an 'in' for an opportunity to tell people about what you do.

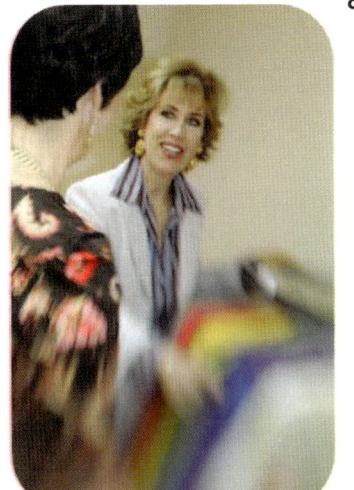

Once you have built up a client base you can move on to more traditional marketing options – internet sites, blogs, in person promotions, flyers, free demonstrations, etc. Use the worksheet attached here to plan your marketing efforts.

The marketing and business promotion worksheets have examples already listed to give you planning ideas. Before you start your *Color Analysis/ Color Consulting* Business you need to work through the following:

1) **Strategic Alliance Spreadsheet** – use this to target business alliances who will help you grow your business by sending you referrals. Explore your existing contacts for referral possibilities.

2) **Target Market Spreadsheet** – client markets you will target to get business.

3) **Marketing Timeline** – detail dates for your market projects and stick to them. Goal setting can be a powerful tool for achieving actual results.

4) **Marketing Strategies** (spend the most time with this worksheet) – plan how you will market your services or business.

Be sure to get focused on your brand image and have cards, brochures etc. completed before you venture out in search of clients.

STRATEGIC ALLIANCE WORKSHEET

Use this planner to list the businesses in your area that can help you gain clients. Once you have determined who you will be aligned with to help you grow your business, contact the business owner and ask to meet with them. Be sure to have your menu of services in brochure format to review with them and always follow up appointments with thank you cards.

When you are searching for alliances remember to target only those businesses that are a good match for you and that can bring you the clients you want to work with.

Alliance Business Name	Service	Contact Name	Address City, State Zip	Phone Number	Email Address	Notes
Hair Pro	Salon	Sandy		5052222222		
Happy Feet	Shoes	Dee				
Junior League	My target market	President of membership				
Women's Networking	Business group				wn@ma.com	

TARGET MARKET WORKSHEET

Identify your ideal client and you improve your chances of attracting the kinds of women, and men, you want to work with. This worksheet asks you to identify who you will be working with, what services you will be offering, how much time you will spend on each project and how much you will charge. This worksheet helps you focus on the income you will be producing in your first year. I've provided a few examples:

Target Client (who do I want to work with)	Product or service to be delivered	How much to charge	How many times per week	Per Month?	Per Year?	$ TOTAL
Lawyers	*Color Consulting*	*$300 for 3 hours*		*1*	*12*	*$3600*
Executives	*Personal Shopping Trip*	*$500 for 3 hours*		*1*	*12*	*$6000*
Celebrities	*Closet Edit Shopping Trip*					
Politicians	*Seminar "How Color Influences Your...."*					
Hair Salons	*Group event*					

MARKETING STRATEGIES FOR YOUR BUSINESS

You may find that you are marketing your products and services to almost everyone you meet. And you should be. This is how you grow a successful business - by letting everyone know who and what you are as a company. This list gives you concrete methods of marketing your business in ways you might not have thought about. Try working through this list on a daily basis and watch your business boom.

Direct Contact or Follow Up	Completed/ Date
Cold calling	
Warm calling - (people you know)	
In person or appointments	
Personal letters and emails	
Announcement cards or letter	
Nice to meet you notes	
Sending articles or web links	
Extending invitations	
Reminder postcards	
Newsletters, e-zines, blogs	
E-mail auto-response and broadcasts	
Network and Referral Building	
Attending meetings and seminars	
Developing referral partners	
Participating in online communities	
Lunch or coffee with contacts	
Staying in touch with former clients	
Volunteering or community service	
Sharing information and resources	
Collaborations and strategic alliances	
Swapping contacts	
Leads groups	
Giving referrals	

Public Speaking	
Hosting meetings	
Serving on panels	
Making presentations	
Giving classes or workshops	
Radio shows	
Writing and Publicity	
Writing articles and tips	
Writing a column	
Publishing a blog	
Being quoted in the media	
Sending press releases	
New product/ service announcements	
Website link	
Getting interviewed	
Promotional Events	
Trade shows	
Free demos or workshops	
Open house or reception	
Co-sponsored events	
Organize your own networking lunch etc.	
Radio show	
Internet	
Website	
Search engine optimizing	
Pay per click	
Banner ads	
E-blasts	
E-news, e-zines	
Podcast/ vid-cast	
Virtual events	
Skype conferencing	

Traditional Advertising	
Newspaper	
Color display ads	
Organizations directories	
Direct mail	
Flyers	
Radio ads	
OTHER:	

SETTING YOUR FEES

How you set your fees is entirely up to you. I can only offer you a few suggestions. Every Color Consultant has a different fee structure. Some will charge per project, some by the hour and others charge for group events. Decide your fees based on your yearly expenses and divide that number by the hours you want to work per day. This should give you a good estimate of the money you need to earn to cover your business expenses.

Formula for Setting an Hourly Fee

Cost of Doing Business for One Year = $50,000

÷ Hours I Want to Work Per Year (300) = $166 per hour

Or charge a flat fee. A good color consultant starts at $275 per hour. The more experience you have and the more clients you get, the higher your fees should go. Don't price yourself out of the market, however. Do get paid what you deserve, remembering that even when working with high end clients, you cannot price gouge. A good rule of thumb on fees: reasonable + fair = return customers.

Always have a professionally printed invoice, with your logo, address and contact information, made out for the client when your service to her is complete.

SAMPLE COLOR ANALYSIS SERVICES AND FEE STRUCTURE

SERVICE	DESCRIPTION	TIME	FEE
Color Analysis and Custom Fan Creation	Test drapes to find skin-tone temperature	3 hours	$175 per hour
Makeup Application and Lesson	Using client inherent colors create a custom makeup chart	2 hours	$400
Shopping Trip	Accompany client on a personal shopping trip	2 hours	$500

Chapter 5 - Articles and Forms

I have included a few articles you can give to your clients. You can customize these by adding your logo and business details. The business forms are also for your use to customize or not. Eventually you'll want to create your own forms with details pertinent to your color analysis sessions.

Articles

Warm or Cool Cheat Sheet

Use this to give clients an idea of what the color analysis process is about. She may have more questions for you once she reads through this.

The Best Colors to Wear for Business Meetings or Lunches

Detailed information about how color can affect one's interactions with friends and colleagues. Color psychology is another field of study and I recommend you read more about it. A good article on the subject is available free at ***www.pantone.com.***

Create a Personal Palette - article about how to identify clients inherent colors.

The Power of Color in Your Wardrobe - tips to help clients identify power colors in clothing.

Forms

Instruction List For Client - prepare your client pre-consultation.

Client Application - use at your first meeting.

Color Quiz - first steps toward determining clients color.

WARM OR COOL?   cheat sheet

- If your skin tone has more yellow, peach, cream then you are warm.

- If your skin tone has more blue, olive or red then you are cool based.

- It is possible, but rare, to be in between; in which case you can wear both cool and warm colors.

- If you are warm toned then everything you wear should have a yellow undertone to it.

- If you are cool toned then your best colors have blue undertones.

Colors can be:

- light/ pale = more white added to the color
- muted/ toasted = black is added
- deep/intense = even more black is added

There are also three levels of contrast to a person's coloring:

Low contrast – very little difference in color between eyes, hair and skin: (Gabrielle/ Desperate Housewives) *Eva Longoria*.
Medium contrast – slight difference in eye, skin and hair color, (Lynette Scavo/ Housewives) *Felicity Huffman*.
High Contrast – Definite contrast between eye, skin and hair color, (Bree van de Kamp/ Housewives) *Marcia Cross*.

PSYCHOLOGY OF COLORS

The Best Colors to Wear for Business Meetings or Lunches (with colleagues or clients)

1. **Black** = power
2. **Navy Blue** = trustworthiness
3. **Royal Blue** = sends out signals of goodwill
4. **Deep Gray** = projects success and strength
5. **Camel** or shades of **Brown** = appears non-threatening, stable, supportive and reliable
6. **Terra-cotta** or **brick** = projects warmth and sensuality
7. **Blue Reds** = indicate warmth, vitality

Colors to Wear When Promoting or Selling a Product

1. **True Blue** or **lighter shades of blue** inspire trust
2. **Orange** is friendly and appeals to all
3. **Yellow** is cheerful and stimulating
4. Blue based **pinks** calm and inspire others

Colors of the Fashion Conscious

1. **Lipstick Red** = implies strength and authority
2. **Fuchsia** = vivaciousness and dynamism
3. **Deep Purple** = indicates creativity and artistic power
4. **Lilac** = spiritual
5. **Muted and clear orange** = warmth and earthiness
6. **Raspberry** = to appear friendly and intelligent
7. **Celadon** = calming and elegant

Create a Personal Palette

We're in the habit of thinking in simplistic terms. We say to ourselves, "I have blue eyes" or we say "I have brown hair." But our coloring is so much more complex than that!

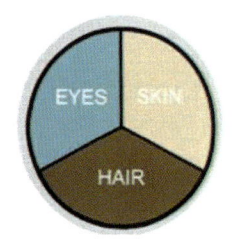

In order to discover your deeper levels of complexity, take a mirror and go either outside or to a large window where you can see your reflection under strong indirect sunlight conditions.

First, identify your **high visibility colors** by taking a close look at your skin, hair, and eyes. Beginning with your eyes, identify **all** of the colors you see. Our eyes are never a single color but are made up of a mosaic of different hues and shades. Write down all of the color variations you see.

Next, look at your hair and repeat this process. Look for the very lightest tones, the mid-tones and the darkest tones. Hair is almost always darker toward the nape of the neck and lighter at the crown and around the face. Make a list of all of the colors you find in your hair.

Finally, repeat this process a third time but this time, look closely at your skin tones. Look for the range of shades from light to dark and also look for the underlying *blush* tones. Make a list of all the colors you see. Be as descriptive and specific as you can. It helps to have a white sheet of paper (or swatch of white fabric) under your hand to help identify your skin tones.

When you have completed this exercise you will have identified your **high visibility colors** (also known as "inherent colors"). These are the colors that reflect your personal color palette. These are colors you can use to form the backbone of your wardrobe and these are colors that will help make you stand out from the crowd. The next time you go shopping take this list of colors with you and use it to guide your purchases. You will be delighted to discover that when your wardrobe repeats the colors of your personal palette **you instantly become more visible.**

The Power of Color in Your Wardrobe

In today's fast-paced world, using color effectively in your wardrobe can determine your position in your company. Use these tips to identify your power colors and implement them into your wardrobe for business success. There are several factors to consider when determining your colors:

Determine if You Have a Warm or Cool Palette

It is relatively easy to determine whether you have a warm or cool palette based on what colors look best on you. If you tend to lean towards earth colors, such as bronzes, gold, earth greens, mochas, browns, and ivories, you most likely have a warm skin tone. If you have a cool skin tone, you may look best in jewel tones, such as emerald green or royal blue.

Or you can use metals as a tool. Pick up some metallic fabric at a local craft store. Stand in front of a mirror in natural light and hold the gold, then the silver fabric next to your face, looking to see which one makes your face 'light up.' If the silver makes your face light up, you are most likely cool-toned. If the gold makes your face light up, you are most likely warm-toned.

Now that you know whether you are a warm or cool-toned, you are equipped to select the colors that will help you turn your drab wardrobe into a power wardrobe.

Plan Your Message with Color

As a successful professional, everyday you probably plan your day and what you want to accomplish with your time. Give the same consideration when planning your attire.

- Ask yourself what is the visual message you want to convey today with your image.
- Is it important today that you get noticed?
- Is it credibility that you mostly want to instill today?

- Or is today the day that you have decided that conveying friendliness and approachability is key?
- Whatever your goal for today, recognize it starts with the colors you select.

Know What Your Colors Are Saying

Each color, of course, comes in many different shades – some are muted, which means the shade has more gray in it, or they are tinted, which means the shade has more white in it. That said, certain colors do convey specific psychological messages overall. For example, red is the color to wear when you want to get attention and appear confident and powerful. For women, a red jacket or suit works really well for this purpose. For a man, using red as an accent color in a tie or pocket handkerchief will still convey the same message with less flair.

Beware of Black

It is also said that the darker the color the more powerful you appear. However, recognize that black can be perceived as intimidating and that may not be what you are after. Although in many industries black is a staple of executive wardrobes, keep in mind that not everyone looks good in black. For some people all you will see is the suit, and not the man or woman. Be sure black accents your appearance rather than overpowers it.

Do Own a Dark Suit

If black is not for you, recognize you still need a dark suit to convey dependability and reliability. Chocolate brown or dark navy blue can be excellent choices. By the way, navy blue, and dark gray are thought to convey professionalism and trustworthiness.

Get a Second Opinion

As an executive you realize the value of hiring a professional. While you may figure out your best colors on your own, an objective professional can be an excellent resource, or at least provide a valuable second opinion. Sometimes we like a color or think it looks good on us based on a past positive association with that color. For example, you may have a soft pink dress that your favorite aunt gave you when she took you on a special trip. Even though it is not the right color for you, you are still drawn to wear it. You may not even be consciously aware that a past positive association with that color is the reason.

Hire a professional image consultant to determine the colors that best suit you. And, if you had your colors done more than ten years ago, or if you have changed your hair color, it is time to get them done again.

There is a lot more to say about color. Make the commitment to yourself to learn more and explore the role color plays in your wardrobe. Apply some of the ideas here to support you in sending the message you want in every work situation. By incorporating the power of color into your wardrobe, you may see dynamic changes in how you are perceived by others in the workplace, and you are more likely to get the results you want every day.

Client Instruction List

Give your client this information sheet prior to her appointment with you.

In preparation of your initial **color consultation** with _____ please review the following.

- Plan to spend 2 hours for your initial color analysis consultation.

- Dress comfortably in loose fitted clothing. You will be sitting in a chair for most of the time.

- Do not wear makeup and don't worry about how your face looks! We will be trying makeup on you during your session.

- Do not wear nail polish. You will get a chance to see which colors look the best on you - including nail polishes.

- Wear your hair down. If you color your hair schedule your visit with your consultant when you have 1/2 inch of root re-growth. This allows us to accurately see your natural hair color and helps us diagnose your underlying color temperature.

- Bring a few pieces of clothing from your wardrobe that are in a color you are not sure suits you. We will review this at the end of your consultation.

- This is **you** time so please don't bring your cell phone, kids or pets with you!

- Don't buy any new clothes until after your color analysis. Likewise makeup, hair color and nail polish!

If you have any questions prior to your appointment please call_____.

Thank you. We look forward to seeing you soon.

CLIENT APPLICATION

NAME:

ADDRESS:

CITY / STATE/ ZIP

CELL PHONE:_____ **HOME PHONE**:_____

EMAIL ADDRESS_____

What is your profession?

How did you hear about us?

Why are you here today?   Fee discussed?

Please write a few words about why you want a color analysis. Let us know what you like and don't like to wear and explain what you hope to achieve from your session today.

Thank you. Please be sure your makeup is removed before your session.

Color Analysis Questionnaire

First Name_____ Last Name_____
Address: _____ City_____ State____ Zip_____
Phone_____ Email_____

1) Describe your facial skin coloring:

Pale and clear
Fair with freckles
Rosy (cheeks with a pink tinge)
Ruddy (spots and colors)
Tanned with golden highlights
Dark with red cheeks
Dark with golden cheeks
Other:

2) Looking at your face in the mirror; how would you describe your overall skin tone?

Clear and Bright
Soft and Muted
Cool and Rosy
Warm and Golden
Light and Fair
Deep and Rich

3) When sun-tanning (with or without sunscreen) does your skin:

Burn easily
Tan slowly
Tan fast

4) What is your natural hair color?

Ash (dirty blond)
Blond
Gray
Brown
Black
Red
Auburn
Other:

5) Describe the color or of your eyes:

Blue
Green
Hazel
Brown
Violet
Other:

6) What color are the small flecks of color in your irises?

White
Black
Rust
Yellow
Deep Blue

7) Go to your makeup bag, find your favorite lipstick color and write the name and brand here:

8) Which shade of lipstick do you prefer

Pink
Red
Coral
Beige
Clear - both

9) What do you have more of in your jewelry box silver or gold?

10) Which colors would you wear if you could only choose three:

Coral, Buttermilk and Bronze
Charcoal, Dusty Rose, Turquoise
Ivory, Tomato Red, Turquoise
Lemon Yellow, Fuchsia, Mint Green

11) What ethnic background are you? Describe.

12) What color is your car?

13) What is your FAVORITE color?

Notes:

2D/3D = EZ©

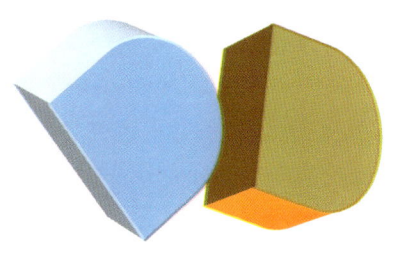

COLOR ANALYSIS CONSULTANT

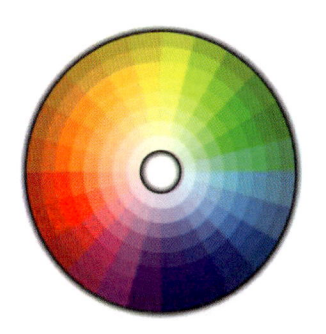

Training and Certification Program

Presented by Gillian Armour, AICI CIP
Certified Color Analyst

2D/3D=EZ© Color Analysis Consultant Training & Certification

As a successful color analyst I've had the great pleasure of introducing hundreds of clients to the joys of color. Clients discovering their best colors undergo irreversible transformations. They go from dressing "yeow" to dressing "wow." I get such joy watching this transformation happen and you will too. Train with me at my color studio and learn the easy Warm / Cool way to complete color determination, color analysis and proper diagnosis. You will learn interactively on live models and will practice painting skin tones. We review Munsell's Color Theory book (the father of color analysis) so you get an education about the origins of color in our world.

I have several color analysis certifications in specializations ranging from ethnic skin tone analysis to flow color analysis. I have practiced color analysis for years and successfully analyzed hundreds of clients. The systems I used in the past were based on the 4, 8 or 12 seasonal color analysis methods (Spring Summer, Autumn, Winter/ low-contrast, high-contrast/ deep, light, bright, clear etc. and etc.). These seasonal systems were quite often confusing for my clients and students - and one day I asked myself "Why are seasonal terms used to identify a person's coloring when in nature there are only **TWO** underlying degrees of temperature (warm and cool)?" I wondered what it would be like to have a simple way to analyze clients, one that would give them a broad range of color options to wear.

Because I wanted a system that was easy to train and easy to explain I simplified my teaching method into a system I call **2D/3D=EZ©** (**two degrees** of color in **three dimensional** views equals **easy**) in the hope that students can better understand how color is analyzed and can better communicate that with their clients. My system simplifies color analysis into degrees of temperature: **WARM** and **COOL**. After all, there are only two color degrees in nature and in the world of color. A client is either warm based or cool based in her skin tone. Simple.

That said, we don't teach "one size fits all" color theory, instead we train your "eye" so that you can analyze an individual's color composition correctly. Far too many trainers neglect this crucial part of color training; at **Fashion Image Institute** we steep you in the science of color analysis so that you become an expert, not just a facilitator of someone's product line.

2D/3D=EZ© Color Analysis Consultant training puts you in the experts chair as a **Certified Color Analyst**. Our 3 day **2D/3D=EZ© Color Analysis Consultant Training** costs $1799 (that's just 3 clients when you consult) and includes Professional Certification, Drapes, Manuals and Books. After you have taken this course, passed all the requirements and completed your first successful color analysis you will be ready to start your own lucrative and exciting **COLOR ANALYSIS BUSINESS**.

All of the following are included in the course:

25 Lesson Modules (combined equal over 24 hours of instruction):

1. Munsell's Color Theory
2. Science of Color
3. History of Color
4. Psychology of Color
5. History of Color Analysis Profession
6. Color Paint Pigment Matching
7. Drape system training
8. **2D/ 3D=EZ©** Color Analysis
9. Custom Color Fan Creation
10. Hair Color Swatches to Determine Hair Shade
11. Skin Coloring Variations
12. Skin Pigmentation
13. Historical Migrations Pertaining to Skin Coloration
14. Contrast in Skin Coloring (Low, Medium, High)
15. Makeup Choices
16. **2D/ 3D=EZ©** Color Books
17. Pantone® Color Predictions
18. Color Prediction and Research
19. How to do a Color Consultation with Clients –Caucasian Origin
20. How to do a Color Consultation with Clients –African Origin
21. How to do a Color Consultation with Clients –Asian Origin
22. How to do a Color Consultation with Clients –Latin Origin
23. Online Hair and Makeup Sessions for Clients
24. Color Coordination in Clothing
25. Color Impact in Film, Fashion and Style and Dress
26. Marketing Your Color Analysis Business
27. Online Color Analysis Web Templates for your business
28. Online Hair Analysis Web Templates for your business
29. Final Exam 45 questions, 1 essay

Additional tools included in the cost of this course:

- A Set of Warm and Cool Color Analysis Drapes ($275 value) to use with your clients
- A Set of Neutral and Metallic Color Analysis Drapes ($75 value)
- Skin Tone Color Examples
- Hair Color Swatches
- Munsell's Color Theory

Recommended Reading (these books will be reviewed during the course)
Color Me Beautiful's Looking Your Best by Mary Spillane ($17.95)
More Alive with Color by Leatrice Eiseman ($19.99)
Color Index by Jim Krause ($24.99)

DAILY CURRICULUM

Schedule	Modules	Times
Day 1 Curriculum	1. Munsell's Color Theory 2. Science of Color 3. History of Color 4. Psychology of Color 5. History of Color Analysis Profession 6. Color Paint Pigment Matching 7. Drape system training 8. **2D/ 3D=EZ©** Color Analysis System 9. Custom Color Fan Creation 10. Hair Color Swatches to Determine Hair Shade 11. Skin Coloring Variations	9am to 12:30pm Lunch 1pm to 5pm
Day 2 Curriculum	1. Skin Pigmentation 2. Historical Migrations Pertaining to Skin Coloration 3. Contrast in Skin Coloring (Low, Medium, High) 4. Makeup Choices 5. **2D/ 3D=EZ©** Color Analysis Books 6. Pantone® Color Predictions 7. Color Prediction and Research 8. How to do a Color Consultation with Clients –Caucasian Origin 9. How to do a Color Consultation with Clients –African Origin 10. How to do a Color Consultation with Clients –Asian Origin 11. How to do a Color Consultation with Clients –Latin Origin 12. Online Hair and Makeup Sessions for Clients	9am to 12:30pm Lunch 1pm to 5pm
Day 3 Curriculum	1. Color Coordination in Clothing 2. Color Impact in Film, Fashion and Style and Dress 3. Marketing Your Color Analysis Business 4. Final Exam	9am to 12:30pm Lunch 1pm to 5pm

Students will be required to pass the final exam with a score of 85% or greater. Learning outcomes and course evaluations need to be completed along with your testimonial regarding your experience with this course before diploma and certification are awarded.

During the course students will be required to successfully complete one color analysis, create skin color fans using paints and color analyze a digital image online.

One essay on the topic of the color analysis process will be completed during the final exam.

Examples of Learning Outcomes for students completing this course:

Upon completion of this course students will be able to:

1. Evaluate The History Of Color Analysis Methods In The USA
2. Discuss The Career Of The Color Analyst
3. Identify Historic Color Theory's
4. Describe Munsell's Color Theory
5. Illustrate The Science Of Color
6. List The Psychological Components Of Color
7. Process Color Analysis Questionnaire With The Model Client
8. Discuss Skin Color Variations Of Migration Patterns
9. Define The Color Wheel
10. Give Examples Of Complementary Colors
11. Give Examples Of Split Complementary Colors
12. Give Examples Of Tertiary Colors
13. Identify Gray Scale
14. Produce A Gray Scale Chart
15. Produce A Hand Painted Personal Palette
16. Discuss Color Draping Systems
17. Introduce The TWO DEGREES OF COLOR
18. Introduce The THREE DIMENSIONS OF COLOR **2D/3D=EZ**©
19. Analyze How Skin Contrast (Low, Medium Or High) Is Determined
20. Paint Skin Tones To Match Personal Skin Coloring
21. Understand How Pigments Are Created
22. Analyze Skin Tone Based On Underlying Skin Components
23. Review What Hue, Chroma And Value Are
24. Describe **2D/3D=EZ**© Use Of Draping Materials
25. List The Drape Colors For Each Degree
26. Produce Sketches Of Color Wheel In The **2D/3D=EZ**© Systems
27. Review Pantone® Color Systems
28. Name The Neutral And Jewel Color Drapes And Their Uses
29. Process A Color Analysis Using A Model
30. Practice Doing A Color Analysis On Themselves
31. Define The Color Temperature Of A Model Client
32. Create A **2D/3D=EZ**© Color Fan For The Model Client
33. Define Hair Color Differences
34. Identify Hair Color Via Online Analysis
35. Write And List The Steps Involved In A **2D/3D=EZ**© Color Analysis
36. Determine Skin, Hair And Eye Contrast In Model Client
37. Identify Correct Cosmetic Choices For Model Client
38. Illustrate A Makeup Chart By Color

39. Review The Fabric And Pattern Choices For Model Client
40. Discuss Color Prediction And Research In Fashion
41. Identify **2D/3D=EZ**© Coloring In Digital Images
42. Review Color Coordination In Clothing
43. Practice The Four Steps To Successful Color Coordination
44. Evaluate Color Impact In Film
45. Evaluate Color Impact In Fashion
46. Evaluate Color Impact In Styling
47. Evaluate Color Impact In Fashion Design
48. Evaluate Color Impact In Dress
49. Discuss Marketing Your Color Analysis Business
50. Produce A One Page Business Plan
51. Give Examples Of Business Forms To Use
52. Process All Strategic Marketing Worksheets
53. Process Target Market Plans
54. Produce Your Business Marketing Plans
55. Demonstrate Understanding Of Color Analysis For Interiors
56. Write An Essay To Demonstrate Understanding Of The Color Wheel

This concludes the course description, curriculum and expected learning outcomes information.

Use the following application to reserve your space in our next class and get trained to do **2D/3D=EZ**© Color Analysis sessions.

Thank you for your interest in our successful program. We look forward to training you for success in this exciting, rewarding and creatively satisfying career.

APPLICATION

We would like to know about your fashion background so please take a moment to tell us about yourself:

Your name: _____

and address (city, state, zip) _____

Your email: _____

Your website: _____

Phone (home and cell) _____

Your fashion background (or experience in a similar field):

_____

_____

_____

_____

Why do you want to be a **2D/3D=EZ© COLOR ANALYSIS CONSULTANT**?

_____

_____

_____

_____

In order to secure your space in class we require a deposit. You are required to pay for the course in its entirety prior to starting. Once we accept your application for enrollment and your deposit you will be emailed a confirmation receipt. Deposits are non-refundable should you decide not to attend the session you have register for.

Payment via Paypal can be made online or visit our website **www.gillianarmour.com** and register on the calendar page for the month of your class.

Email a copy of this application to **contact@fashionimageinstitute.com**

Name on card: _____

Card number and expiration date: _____

Secure 3 digit code: _____

Please sign and date here: _____

By signing this agreement you commit to attending the following course (list the date of your course, the subject and location): _____

_____

This course is offered in accordance with the Association of Image Consultants (A.I.C.I) core competencies for Image Consultant Certification. Once students have completed the course requirements they will be eligible and prepared to begin study for the First Level Certification (FLC) offered by A.I.C.I. We strive to prepare you and your portfolio for successful acceptance into FLC designation.

This course is currently in the process of CEU approval with AICI. Students taking this course will be presented with official **Color Analysis Consultant Certification** and will be able to start consulting with clients immediately. Students will be required to:

- Pass three exams, a final exam and essay
- Process a color analysis on a client
- Complete the ***Participant Training Evaluation***
- Complete the course evaluation form
- Write a testimonial about the course experience and
- Submit a portfolio of projects completed in class

Please feel free to call us if you have any further questions about the course.
You can reach us at (415) 230-0015 or via email at contact@fashionimageinstitute.com

ABOUT THE AUTHOR

Fashion Journalist, TV Presenter and Celebrity Fashion Stylist, Gillian Armour is the CEO and founder of **Fashion Image Institute**. Her company develops online educational programs on personal style and professional development. Gillian has put her fashion skills to good use by training other experts in the image, style and fashion fields. She hosts the award winning cable television series - Dream Makeover. She is the designer behind Couture Jewels and the author of seven books on style, image, career and color.

Gillian is a Certified Image Professional (CIP) through the prestigious **Association of Image Consultants**. She is a Certified Personal Shopper and Certified Personal Trainer. She has transformed hundreds of clients over the years. Gillian is one of only ninety three CIP's in the USA. She also helms a teaching studio in San Francisco, California in the heart of the Union Square fashion district.

Clients from the real estate, hotel, financial and legal industries, along with the government and military, have used Gillian Armour Image Consulting to establish appropriate levels of dress and grooming critical to business relations. While much of the consulting focuses on individual work, Gillian Armour Image Consulting also offers seminars and workshops for companies looking to set a standard, establish a dress code or create a signature workforce appearance. Her website **www.imagetalks.com** provides customizable programs for national speakers. Gillian is a Professional Member of the National Speakers Association and speaks regularly on topics of executive appearance, communication and behavior.

In 2007, Gillian formed **Best Dressed**[sm] to help men, women and teens from economically challenged backgrounds enter the workforce by offering free of charge makeover and wardrobe services to qualified clients actively seeking employment. **Best Dressed**[sm] is a 501(c)3 nonprofit organization.

Websites:

www.gillianarmour.com
www.fashionimageinstitute.com
www.imagetalks.com

Resources:

Pantone Color - www.pantone.com
Color Books - www.amazon.com
Color Guides - www.colorguides.net
Hair Swatches - www.wigs.com
Lab Coats - www.labwear.com
Color Analysis Tool, Fans and Drapes - www.fashionimageinstitute.com
Color jpegs images - www.fashionimageinstitute.com

Contact:

(415) 230-0015
email: contact@fashionimageinstitute.com

Books by Gillian Armour Available at www.amazon.com and other retailers

Mastering the Art of Business Image
Fashion Stylist - a How To Guide
Fashion Silhouette Illustrations - Flatter Your Body Shape
The Elite Personal Shopper
How to Do an Image Consult
Mastering the Art of Dressing Well
Face Design and Makeup

NOTES

NOTES

Made in the USA
Lexington, KY
22 March 2012